TRAPPED

AT THE

BEDSIDE

Unexpected Paths to Your Unique Purpose Within Bedside Nursing

WORKBOOK INCLUDED INSIDE

ROBERT MCGEE JR., BSN, RN

TRAPPED AT THE BEDSIDE

Unexpected Paths to Your Unique Purpose Within Bedside Nursing

ACKNOWLEDGMENT

To my editor, Nick Potts at Gold Medal Editing, thank you for seeing what this book could be and helping me get it there. Your patience and honest feedback made this work better than I could have made it alone.

TABLE OF CONTENTS

THE FEELING OF BEING TRAPPED

If you're reading this, you've probably felt it. That nagging sense you're meant for something more in your nursing career. You're not alone in these thoughts.

I'm writing this note to you after spending fourteen years at the bedside. I've worked under every type of leader. Great nurse leaders who keep their teams engaged and push each person to grow in ways that actually fit who they are. Leaders who do just enough to meet their metrics and keep their jobs. And I've seen the kind of blatant favoritism that crushes nurses at the bedside, where staff watch their own aspirations become unreachable under a leader who's protected by decision makers too proud to admit they made a mistake. Night shift, day shift, charge nurse, travel nurse, float pool—I've done them. And what stands out most? The bedside nurses I've met along the way.

Most of the nurses I started my career with have left the bedside. I said goodbye to so many nurses even before COVID-19 triggered the mass exodus. I believe the pandemic only accelerated what was already happening. I remember my first COVID-19 positive patient. At our facility, the rules were clear: only bedside nurses and respiratory therapists would enter those rooms. PCTs would stand in the hallway passing supplies through the door. Inside, you were completely alone. As the bedside nurse, I became everything. I removed meal trays, hauled out trash and soiled linens, took vital signs, changed patients, and did every single task that was normally shared among the team. Just me, in full PPE, feeling more isolated than I'd ever felt in my career.

The pandemic has come and gone, but the isolation I felt in those COVID rooms has become a mirror for what so many of us experience every single day at the bedside. Feeling alone, trapped, and unsupported. But here's what I believe to be true: What you're experiencing is the tension between the profound impact you're already making and your inability to see how that impact can open new doors.

You have gifts that are uniquely yours—ways of connecting with patients, solving problems, or bringing calm to complexity that nobody else can replicate. But you can't see how those gifts could possibly create a meaningful career path. That's not a career problem. That's a vision problem. And vision problems can be fixed. Our vision shapes our purpose because it tells us where we are going. When we do not know where we are going, we move without direction, or worse, we become hopeless.

If one idea in this book helps you see a clearer path forward in your nursing career, I'll call that a win. But if that idea becomes the key that unlocks a career path aligned with your authentic self, this book will have done what it was meant to do. Speaking of career paths, I have a question for you.

What if everything we've been told about your nursing career path is only half the story?

Your unique purpose isn't something you need to find by escaping your current role. It was already with you before you clocked in for your first shift, and it's exactly what will guide you through whatever challenges you're facing right now. Your unique purpose and your bedside experience have been preparing you for something bigger all along. I believe true success happens when you're doing exactly what you were created to do.

The bedside teaches you something about the human condition that you can't learn anywhere else. Your proximity to the human struggle builds your capacity to manage pressure in ways most people never develop. Working at the bedside also shapes you into an advocate, whether you planned it or not. You speak up because something matters more than staying quiet.

But there's a skill embedded in all of this that often goes unnoticed: We've learned to read what's unsaid—to detect the micro-signals in a patient's face, tone, or body language that reveal what lab values and algorithms miss. We know how to sense when something is "off" before the data catches up, to hear the fear beneath the casual question, to notice the family dynamic that will determine whether a care plan succeeds or fails. It's a form of human pattern recognition that can't be automated. And in a world where artificial intelligence will handle more routine tasks, this ability to interpret unmeasurable data matters more than ever.

We don't just read the room. We know how to translate what we sense into actionable data that predicts outcomes, bridging the gap between human intuition and measurable impact. This is what bedside nursing gives us: superpowers. Superpowers that are desperately needed not just in patient rooms, but in healthcare leadership, policy development, technology innovation, education, research, and countless other areas where the patient perspective is missing or misunderstood. Your path forward isn't about outgrowing bedside nursing but leveraging your bedside experience as the foundation for something uniquely yours. But first, I need you to consider something.

What if you're not actually trapped at the bedside?

This distinction will either frustrate you or free you, depending on how ready you are to hear it. You may feel trapped, but feeling trapped and being trapped are two entirely different realities. What if you're not actually trapped at the bedside? What if you're wandering through a maze? A trap is designed with malicious intent. Traps are meant to capture you and keep you exactly where you are, with no plan for your escape. The trap benefits from your hopeless thoughts of imprisonment. But a maze? A maze serves an entirely different purpose. A maze tests your capacity to navigate complexity. It challenges your ability to stay calm when the path ahead isn't clear. It asks you to trust that forward movement is possible even when you can't see where you're going. A maze doesn't want to keep you—it wants to see if you can find your way through.

Feeling trapped usually means you've hit one of these maze challenges that make it tough to see your options:

> **Career Plateau:** Feeling your current role is no longer challenging or that advancement opportunities within your specialty are limited, leading to questions about long-term professional growth and development.

> **Role Misalignment:** Not finding opportunities that align with your evolving interests, skills, or career goals, or sensing that your talents could be better utilized in different ways within healthcare.

> **Transitional Uncertainty:** Not knowing how to leverage your valuable nursing skills and experience into new roles or specialties, especially when there's a gap between your training and the expanding possibilities within nursing.

Every maze has at least one way out, and most have several. The uncertainty you're feeling right now isn't proof that bedside nursing is a one-way dead end. It's proof that your mind is already reaching for what comes next. The workbook at the back of this book is there to help you bridge that gap, because reading about new pathways and actually finding your way are two very different things. Take a deep breath. You're not trapped. You're at the beginning of something new.

Now, let's take your first step forward together!

YOUR UNIQUE STRUGGLE

CHAPTER ONE

BREAKING FREE STARTS HERE

Recognizing Your Starting Point

Naming your reality gives you the power to change it.

A maze can be intimidating. You see the turns ahead, but no matter how many steps you take, the exit feels far away. You're always in motion, but instead of making meaningful progress, you find yourself circling back to the same frustrations. The bedside maze isn't something that confines you; it's something that prepares you for bigger opportunities. The problem is no one has told you that you should be moving through the maze, so you've been running into dead ends thinking you were trapped at the bedside.

The maze never stays the same. Some shifts, you walk onto the unit and everything clicks. Your patients are stable, your assignments make sense, and you find a rhythm that feels almost effortless. You anticipate needs before the call lights go off. Your charting stays current. You even have a moment to grab your coffee while it's still warm. These are the shifts that remind you why you chose this work.

Then there are the shifts that test every ounce of your resilience. You haven't finished your first assessment before three alarms are beeping, the pharmacy is calling about a clarification, and a family member stops you in the hallway with a list of questions. Tasks multiply faster than you can complete them.

By mid-shift, you're running on adrenaline and muscle memory, wondering how the same job can feel so different from one day to the next. This is the nature of the maze. It expands and contracts. It offers stretches of clarity and then throws obstacles in your path without warning.

Most nurses don't realize that the emotion of feeling trapped rarely comes from one difficult day. It usually sneaks up on you when you mistake a rough patch for your permanent reality. When you can't see a clear path forward in your career, it's natural to think you're stuck in a role that will never grow or change. With this understanding that you're moving through a maze rather than trapped without options, let's identify exactly where you are in your journey. The first step in navigating any maze is recognizing the landmarks that tell you where you've been and where you might be headed.

The Peaks: Moments of Clarity and Strength

Peaks are the moments when the maze feels manageable, when you rise above the demands and clearly remember why you chose this path in the first place. These are the moments when you know, without a doubt, that what you're doing matters. It could be as simple as a patient squeezing your hand and saying, "Thank you for being here," or as profound as recognizing a subtle sign that prevents a patient from rapidly declining.

Sometimes peaks are subtle. They're found in the nod from a coworker that says, "You handled that like a PRO," or the moment you finally get a restless patient to relax. They might seem insignificant to an outsider, but after a long day in the maze, they feel monumental. Peaks don't last forever, and that's okay. They're not about achieving notoriety; they're about gaining perspective. They remind you that you've successfully navigated challenges before and that you have the skills to find your way through whatever comes next.

The Valleys: When the Maze Feels Smothering

For every peak, there's a valley. Valleys are the moments when the walls of the maze feel like they're closing in. The path narrows to a point where you can barely breathe. It's the shift where no matter how hard you try, nothing seems to go right. The patient who was stable takes a turn for the worse. The schedule changes mid-shift, throwing everything off. In moments like these, you second-guess yourself, wondering if you really want to continue doing this.

Valleys make you question your purpose. They make you feel small, like you're just another cog in a system that never stops. You're surrounded by patients, families, and coworkers, but the emotional load makes you feel completely isolated. The hardest part about valleys is that they make you forget the peaks ever existed. They whisper lies like, "You're not a good nurse" and "You're stuck at the bedside." But deep down, you know that's not true.

Recognizing Where You Are

The first step toward finding your way isn't continuing to go through the motions—it's understanding where you are right now. Stop and ask yourself:

> When was the last time you felt like you were standing on a peak? What made you feel strong, capable, and connected to your purpose?

> When was the last time you felt like you were in a valley? What made you feel overwhelmed, unsure, or disconnected?

> What part of your daily work feels like you're moving, but not really getting anywhere?

The maze is an unavoidable part of bedside nursing, but how you navigate it makes all the difference. When you find yourself in a valley, recognizing that it's temporary gives you the resilience to keep moving forward. You can grant yourself permission to pause, reach out for support, or take one meaningful step that shifts your mindset. When you're experiencing a peak, truly acknowledging your progress helps you build confidence instead of dismissing it as simply doing your job.

Identifying where you are doesn't require you to predict what's coming next or have all the answers mapped out. It means you're consciously aware of where you currently stand, which gives you clarity to make intentional decisions about where to head next. This awareness transforms you from someone who feels lost in the maze to someone who's actively choosing their path through it, and that choice is the first step toward discovering the unique purpose that's been waiting for you all along.

REFLECTION EXERCISE:
MAPPING YOUR MAZE

Let's slow down for a second and think:

- What does your maze look like right now?
- What's one step you can take today to remind yourself that you're still moving, even if you can't see the exit?

CHAPTER TWO

THE POWER TO PIVOT

Using Change to Break Free

A pivot is not weakness—it's
wisdom in motion.

Change doesn't ask for our permission. It happens whether you're ready or not. Healthcare moves forward constantly, bringing new leaders with fresh visions, transforming familiar workflows you mastered last month into obsolete processes the next.

Even when the goal is improving patient care, change often feels like an inconvenience rather than progress.

It's like walking a familiar path in the maze, only to find the ground has shifted beneath your feet. The maze of bedside nursing will continue to evolve, and if you stand still as the ground shifts, you'll only sink deeper into your frustrations.

Redefining Professional Identity Beyond Role Stagnation

Most of us entered nursing with a clear sense of purpose, but somewhere along the way, we began equating professional loyalty with staying put.

We've absorbed this message from countless small moments: the way colleagues talk about the nurse who "abandoned" the unit for a different specialty, the raised eyebrows when someone mentions considering a move, the subtle implication that loyalty means staying exactly where you are. This version of loyalty holds everyone back.

Think about the last time you felt genuinely excited about going to work—not just satisfied or competent, but truly energized. If you can't remember, that's okay. Don't panic.

This is what happens when we mistake staying static for staying loyal. Your value as a nurse isn't determined by how long you've been in the same role. These are the stories we tell ourselves, but they're not serving us or our patients.

The healthcare system needs nurses who refuse to accept "that's just how we've always done it" as a final answer. It needs nurses who look at inefficient processes and think, "There has to be a better way." When you stay stuck because you think it's the noble thing to do, you're not protecting anything valuable. You're preventing something valuable from emerging. Every insight you could have brought to a new environment stays locked away. Every innovation that might have sparked from your unique perspective remains unrealized.

The most patient-centered thing you can do might be to follow your own professional curiosity. Patients don't need martyrs who drag themselves through shifts they've long since outgrown. They need nurses who show up fully engaged, who bring their best selves to work because they're doing work that actually fits who they're becoming. Sometimes the most loyal thing you can do for nursing is to become the nurse you're truly meant to be, even if that means disappointing people who preferred the version of you that was easier to predict.

Why Your Brain Fights Career Evolution

Resistance to change is human nature, especially when you've finally found your rhythm. But when the maze shifts around you, comfort becomes a trap. Your brain, designed to keep you safe, interprets career uncertainty as potential danger.

This isn't a character flaw or personal weakness; it's basic human neurobiology working exactly as designed. Resistance to change shows up in different ways. Maybe you quietly avoid new processes, sticking to old routines that feel safer. Perhaps you find yourself venting to coworkers more than problem-solving, or freezing altogether when change feels too overwhelming to navigate.

Career stagnation, when prolonged, can trigger the chronic stress responses that ultimately manifest as burnout. When we examine change through a neurological lens, fascinating patterns emerge. Research demonstrates that burnout creates distinctive changes in brain anatomy and functioning, particularly affecting the prefrontal cortex, which governs executive functions, abstract thinking, and decision-making (Arnsten & Shanafelt, 2021)[1]. Understanding these neurobiological changes helps explain why burnout makes change feel more difficult—not because of personal weakness, but because chronic stress literally alters brain function.

Yale neuroscientist Amy Arnsten's research reveals that chronic stress weakens the prefrontal cortex while strengthening primitive brain circuits like the amygdala—the region responsible for generating fear and other survival-driven emotions. You can possibly start seeing change as harmful even when it's not (Arnsten, 2009)[2]. This neurobiological reality explains one of the most insidious aspects of burnout: settling into what researchers describe as comfortable discomfort. This occurs when current conditions, while deeply unsatisfying, feel safer than the uncertainty of change. We become accustomed to the familiar ache of exhaustion, the predictable rhythm of overwhelming shifts, the known quantity of our daily struggles.

Neuroplasticity means our brains can literally rewire themselves through consistent, intentional practice. Researchers define it as 'the ability of the nervous system to change its activity in response to intrinsic or extrinsic stimuli by reorganizing its structure, functions, or connections' (Mateos-Aparicio & Rodríguez-Moreno, 2019)[3]. For

---

1 Arnsten, A. F., & Shanafelt, T. D. (2021). Physician distress and burnout: The neurobiological perspective. *Mayo Clinic Proceedings*, 96(3), 763-769. https://pmc.ncbi.nlm.nih.gov/articles/PMC7944649/

2 Arnsten, A. F. T. (2009). Stress signalling pathways that impair prefrontal cortex structure and function. Nature Reviews Neuroscience, 10(6), 410-422. https://doi.org/10.1038/nrn2648

3 Mateos-Aparicio, P., & Rodríguez-Moreno, A. (2019). The impact of studying brain plasticity. *Frontiers in Cellular Neuroscience*, 13, Article 66. https://doi.org/10.3389/fncel.2019.00066

nurses feeling trapped in burnout cycles, neuroplasticity offers genuine hope that change is not only possible but achievable through sustained action.

Breaking free from comfort requires acknowledging that the pain of staying the same will eventually exceed the pain of changing. Movement disrupts this cycle and creates space for new neural pathways to develop.

These new neural pathways don't just help you cope better with your current situation; they create a path to an entirely different future, one that aligns more closely with your authentic purpose.

The Compound Effect of Small Professional Experiments

Let's explore a practical way forward—one that doesn't involve sprinting ahead blindly or staying rooted in frustration. It involves choosing small, intentional steps that help you regain your balance and rebuild your sense of agency. Movement isn't about speed; it's about intention.

Organizational psychologist Karl Weick's research on "small wins" provides a scientifically-backed framework for creating sustainable change. Weick defined small wins as "concrete, complete outcomes of moderate importance" that build momentum over time (Weick, 1984)[4]. His research demonstrates that when problems feel overwhelming, breaking them into smaller, manageable pieces reduces excessive stress and creates opportunities for innovative action.

---

4 Weick, K. E. (1984). Small wins: Redefining the scale of social problems. American Psychologist, 39(1), 40-49. https://doi.org/10.1037/0003-066X.39.1.40

The psychology of small wins operates through several mechanisms. First, small wins reduce the cognitive load required for decision-making, making action feel more manageable. Second, they provide evidence that change is possible, building confidence for larger steps. Third, they create positive feedback loops that reinforce continued progress (Weick, 1984) [5]. So, what does this look like practically? Instead of feeling you need to completely overhaul your career overnight, you might start by having one conversation with a nurse working in a different specialty. Instead of impulsively pursuing an advanced degree, you might attend one nursing workshop about a topic that sparks your curiosity. Instead of leaving bedside nursing altogether, you might volunteer to participate in a quality improvement project. The most valuable aspect of movement involves what it reveals about ourselves.

When we take action, even small action, we gather information about our preferences, strengths, and values that isn't available through reflection alone. This experiential learning becomes crucial for nurses exploring new directions. Movement provides lessons that thinking cannot. We learn by taking action, not by sitting still. You might think you'd hate working in education until you spend an afternoon precepting a new nurse and discover something lights up inside you that's been dormant for months.

Your discomfort with your current situation is your internal signal that you've outgrown your previous path and you're ready for something

---

5 Weick, K. E. (1984). Small wins: Redefining the scale of social problems. American Psychologist, 39(1), 40-49. https://doi.org/10.1037/0003-066X.39.1.40

more aligned with who you're becoming. Your willingness to feel uncomfortable with where you are is actually the first requirement for discovering where you're meant to go next.

Change doesn't mean abandoning everything you've learned. The nurse you are today contains all the wisdom of every patient you've cared for, every crisis you've navigated, every moment you chose compassion over convenience. That wisdom doesn't disappear when you grow; it becomes the foundation for something even more meaningful. Navigating the maze doesn't require dramatic leaps or complete career overhauls. It requires consistent, intentional movement in directions that feel increasingly aligned with your authentic self. Each small action builds upon the previous one, creating momentum that eventually leads to transformation you couldn't have planned at the start of your nursing career.

The freedom you seek begins with starting before you feel ready. The maze will teach you what you need to know, but only if you're willing to move through it instead of waiting for someone to hand you a neatly drawn map.

REFLECTION EXERCISE:
Discovering Your Hidden Values and Unique Approach

♡ Exercise 1: The Values Collision Map

Think of three moments in your nursing career when you felt most frustrated or morally distressed, then identify what core value was being compromised in each situation. Next, identify three moments when you felt most alive and authentic in your practice, noting which values were fully expressed.

♀ Exercise 2: The Patient Story Mirror

Write the stories of a few patients who impacted you most deeply, focusing on the human elements rather than medical details. What touched something inside you about each person? What did you learn about yourself through caring for them?

View these stories as mirrors reflecting your own needs, dreams, and nursing journey. The patients who affect us most deeply often point toward our unique purpose, revealing the aspects of nursing that align with our soul's work.

Bonus Reflection Exercise: Naming Your Next Step

Spend a moment considering the following:

- ♀ What recent change has made you feel disoriented or frustrated?
- ♀ How did you respond—did you resist, adjust, or freeze?
- ♀ What's one small, intentional step you can take today to move forward?

Write down your answers. Naming your experience and your response can help you see your progress more clearly.

CHAPTER THREE

PEAK PERFORMANCE CLUES

Your Sweet Spot at the Bedside

The work that feels easiest often reveals your greatest strength.

Every nurse's maze is unique, shaped by their particular unit, patient population, work schedule, and at-home circumstances. But all nursing mazes share common elements: routine tasks, unexpected emergencies, understaffing, and yes, elevated vantage points where everything suddenly makes sense.

Every maze has internal logic, patterns, and most importantly, elevated points where you can see further and reorient yourself. In nursing, these peaks come in the form of meaningful patient encounters that reconnect you with your purpose and show you possibilities you couldn't see from the ground level.

The Science Behind Why Peaks Matter

Psychologist Mihály Csíkszentmihályi spent decades studying what he termed "flow states"—those moments when we become completely absorbed in an activity, lose track of time, and perform at our optimal level. In his seminal work, he described flow as "a state in which people are so involved in an activity that nothing else seems to matter; the experience is so enjoyable that people will continue to do it even at great cost, for the sheer sake of doing it" (Csíkszentmihályi, 1990)[6]. Research specifically with nurses has identified that "flow situations can be identified through individuals' estimates of perceived challenge and skills" during everyday nursing practice (Persson et al., 2001)[7]. This groundbreaking study found that nurses regularly experience flow states during patient care, particularly when their skills are well-matched to the challenges they face.

What makes this research revolutionary for nurses in the bedside maze is Csíkszentmihályi's discovery that "flow occurred more often during work than free time." Your nursing practice is actually primed for peak experiences—you just need to recognize and cultivate them.

When you experience a peak moment in nursing—your brain undergoes remarkable changes. Research shows that when individuals perceive a balance between the challenges of a task and their own skill

---

[6] Csíkszentmihályi, M. (1990). *Flow: The psychology of optimal experience.* Harper & Row.

[7] Persson, D., Erlandsson, L.-K., Eklund, M., & Iwarsson, S. (2001). Flow situations during everyday practice in a medical hospital ward. Results from a study based on experience sampling method. *BMC Nursing, 10*(3). https://doi.org/10.1186/1472-6955-10-3

levels, they enter an optimal psychological state characterized by deep engagement and a profound sense of fulfillment.

These neurobiological changes create what researchers call "context-triggered flow" and "self-regulated flow." Context-triggered flow happens when your environment naturally creates the conditions for peak experience—like when you find a rhythm in completing tasks during a complex procedure or when you provide exactly what a patient needs in a moment of crisis. Self-regulated flow is even more powerful because it represents your ability to intentionally create conditions for meaningful moments. These two flow states are proof that you can find your footing in the maze, even when everything around you feels unpredictable.

The Three Moments When Clarity Emerges

> **Presence Peaks:** These occur when you're completely focused on a patient during a significant moment—a difficult conversation or a moment of comfort—and everything else around you seems to quiet down. Research confirms what you likely already sense—meaningful encounters create life-changing insights and foster trust, cooperation, and wellbeing for both patients and healthcare professionals (Gustafsson et al., 2013)[8].

How to create them: Choose one patient interaction per shift where you practice complete presence. Put down your phone, make eye

---

[8] Gustafsson, L.-K., Snellman, I., & Gustafsson, C. (2013). The meaningful encounter: Patient and next-of-kin stories about their experience of meaningful encounters in health-care. *Nursing Inquiry, 20*(4), 363-371. https://doi.org/10.1111/nin.12013

contact, and listen with your whole attention. Notice if this changes the quality of the patient encounter and how it makes the rest of your encounters with this patient feel more manageable.

> **Competence Peaks:** These happen when your skills perfectly match the challenge at hand, and you feel the maze working with you instead of against you. Csikszentmihalyi found that flow occurs when there is an optimal balance between the challenge of a task and a person's skill level, along with clear goals and immediate feedback. It usually stretched the person's capacity and provided a challenge to his or her skills".

How to create them: Identify one skill you want to develop or refine. Practice it intentionally during appropriate situations, seeking feedback and gradually increasing the complexity. Notice the satisfaction that comes from growing competence and how it makes challenging situations feel more manageable.

> **Purpose Peaks:** These emerge when you suddenly see the bigger picture of why your work matters—when you realize the impact you're having on patients' lives or witness how your nursing skills make a real difference.

How to create them: At the end of each shift, identify one specific way you made a difference in someone's experience. Write it down. Over time, you'll see patterns of purpose that weren't visible day to day, and these small reminders will help you navigate even the most challenging shifts.

You don't need to know where these peaks will lead. You just need to keep climbing to the next one. One peak may give you a glimpse over the wall of your current situation. The view from each high point reveals new possibilities that weren't visible from below and reminds you that the maze has a purpose—and so do you.

When you feel disoriented and the maze seems impossible, return to these research-backed truths:

> *"Flow occurs more often during work than leisure"*—Your nursing practice is designed for peak experiences.

> *"Meaningful encounters create life-changing moments"*—Every patient interaction has peak potential.

> *"Small wins build momentum for larger transformations"*—Each peak prepares you for bigger movements.

> *"I can intentionally create conditions for flow"*—You have more control than you realize.

> *"The maze feels manageable when I remember my purpose"*—Peaks reconnect you to why you're here.

Peaks often hide in ordinary moments that are easy to overlook. Some of the most powerful are what I call presence peaks, those unexpected connections that emerge simply because you slowed down long enough to see your patient as a whole person.

I experienced one recently with a 71-year-old patient. Through casual conversation, I discovered she had graduated from my high school. Her son was a fire chief at a fire department near where I used to live.

We had both relocated from one big city to this new city, hundreds of miles from where we went to school, yet here we were. In that moment, we established a connection unlike any I'd experienced with other patients that day. She seemed to trust without hesitation every word I spoke from that moment forward. Nothing extraordinary happened. I simply slowed down enough to ask about her life. That small choice created a purpose peak of genuine human connection that reminded me of why our connecting work matters.

Your peaks don't need an audience, and you don't need applause to validate them. The power of a peak lies in how it makes the maze feel manageable again and reminds you that you deserve these moments of reconnection with your professional purpose.

These peaks, whether dramatic or quietly ordinary, reveal that feeling trapped at the bedside isn't a limitation but an opportunity for discovering what makes your nursing practice uniquely meaningful.

Keep climbing. The view gets
better with each elevation.

CHAPTER FOUR

THE VALLEYS OF GROWTH

Learning from the Low Points

A nurse who learns from valleys
rises stronger than one who
only celebrates peaks.

The valleys aren't your enemy—they're your teacher. Finding yourself in a valley while navigating the maze doesn't mean you've lost your way. You don't end up in a valley by sitting on the sidelines. You're in the thick of it because you're showing up and giving everything you've got. Valleys are the battlegrounds where you learn what you're really made of—and if you've made it this far, you've already proven that you're tougher than you think. But let's be real—valleys suck. They're messy, uncomfortable, and sometimes unforgiving. These are the shifts where nothing goes right. You're running low on energy, patience, and answers all at the same time. It's the patient who starts to decline later in your shift after you've been watching them like a hawk. It's the family member who questions your care even though you've poured your heart into their loved one. These moments are when the maze feels the tightest—like the walls are closing in. But valleys aren't dead ends. Valleys strip away the noise and force you to confront what's real. They test your patience, your boundaries, and your belief in yourself. That's exactly why they have the potential to teach you so much.

Valleys are inevitable. The nurse who can handle anything isn't built on easy assignments. Growth lives in the valleys. What if you stopped seeing valleys as setbacks and started seeing them as opportunities? Not in some cheesy "everything happens for a reason" way, but in a way that reminds you that valleys have lessons hidden in the struggle. When you're in the valley, you're face-to-face with your limits—but you're also face-to-face with your strength. Maybe you walked away from those moments feeling defeated. But look at you. You've made it this far. Every step through the maze, every challenge, brings you closer to your next peak.

When you're standing at a high point in a maze, you might feel like you're on top of the world. But valleys offer an entirely different perspective. From the low places, you can often spot openings and pathways that were invisible from above. The crushing realization that bedside nursing isn't what you expected might actually be your first step toward discovering what kind of nurse you were always meant to become. This realization usually doesn't come during our peak experiences.

The Five Valleys Every Bedside Nurse Knows

While every nurse's maze is unique, there are certain valleys that show up with remarkable consistency. If I could sit down with a hundred nurses and ask them to tell me about their lowest moments in nursing, I believe I'd hear the same themes over and over again.

Heartbreaking because it means so many caring, competent nurses go through periods of questioning everything they thought they knew about themselves and their profession. Comforting because it means you're not alone and you're not losing your mind. You look around at your colleagues who seem to have it all together, and you wonder what's wrong with you. Why does that nurse over there seem energized by the same work that's leaving you depleted? Why are you the only one who seems to be struggling with this?

You're not the only one struggling. That nurse who looks like they have everything figured out? They've probably been exactly where you are, or they will be soon. The colleague who seems endlessly patient with difficult patients? They've likely had nights where they questioned whether they had any compassion left. The experienced nurse who makes everything look effortless? Ask them about their first year of nursing, and you'll probably hear a story that sounds remarkably familiar.

The patterns I'm about to describe aren't universal in their timing or intensity, but they're common enough that recognizing them can help you understand that what you're experiencing isn't the end of your nursing career. It's a part of the bedside nursing journey that has valuable lessons to teach, even when those lessons feel like they're being delivered with a sledgehammer rather than a gentle nudge.

The Valley of Feeling Incompetent

This valley typically hits somewhere between six months and two years into your nursing career, just when you thought you were finally getting the hang of things. One day you're feeling confident about your skills, and the next day you're questioning everything you think you know about nursing. Maybe it's the patient whose condition deteriorated on your watch, and you didn't pick up the subtle signs. Maybe it's realizing that the experienced nurse next to you handled a similar situation with an ease that feels impossible to imagine for yourself. Or maybe it's that moment when you realize there's so much about nursing that nursing school never taught you, and you wonder if you'll ever really know enough to do this job well.

This valley of incompetence is actually a sign of growing awareness. Skill acquisition research demonstrates that awareness of one's limitations at the novice stage is essential for advancing through subsequent levels of competence toward true expertise (Dreyfus & Dreyfus, 1986)[9].

The fact that you can see the gaps in your knowledge and skills means you're developing the clinical judgment to recognize them.

---

[9] Dreyfus, H. L., & Dreyfus, S. E. (1986). *Mind over machine: The power of human intuition and expertise in the era of the computer.* Free Press.

The Valley of Moral Distress

This might be the most heartbreaking valley of all: the growing awareness that you can't always provide the care you know your patients need. You went into nursing to help people, to make a difference, to be part of healing. But the reality of healthcare systems, insurance limitations, staffing shortages, and family dynamics means that sometimes the right thing for your patient isn't the thing you're able to do. You watch a patient suffer because pain medication orders are inadequate, but the physician won't return your calls. You know a patient needs more time and attention than you can give because you're responsible for too many other patients. You see family members making decisions that aren't in the patient's best interest, but your hands are tied by legal and ethical constraints.

This valley teaches you about the complexity of healthcare and your role within larger systems. It also teaches you to distinguish between the care you can control and the factors you cannot.

The Valley of Physical Exhaustion

There comes a point in many nurses' careers when the tiredness changes. It's no longer the kind of tiredness that goes away after a good night's sleep or a few days off. It's a bone-deep exhaustion that follows you home, affects your relationships, and makes you dread the sound of your alarm clock. Your feet hurt in new ways. Your back aches randomly. You find yourself getting sick more often, and when you do get time off, you spend most of it recovering rather than enjoying life.

This valley teaches you about the importance of self-care, boundaries, and sustainability in your career. It forces you to confront the reality that nursing is physically and emotionally demanding work that requires intentional strategies for preservation and renewal.

The Valley of Lost Empathy

Perhaps nothing is more alarming to a caring nurse than the gradual realization that you're becoming numb to your patients' experiences. The stories that used to move you to tears now feel routine.

The family members who are clearly struggling with fear and grief start to feel more like obstacles to your efficiency than human beings deserving of compassion.

You catch yourself being impatient with patients who are demanding or difficult. You realize you're going through the motions of caring without actually feeling much of anything.

This valley is terrifying because empathy and compassion feel so central to who you are as a nurse. What you're experiencing is what researchers call compassion fatigue—the emotional exhaustion that results from prolonged empathic engagement with suffering (Figley, 2002)[10].

Rather than accepting emotional distancing as inevitable, the key is learning the difference between protective emotional boundaries and harmful disconnection.

---

[10] Figley, C. R. (2002). Compassion fatigue: Psychotherapists' chronic lack of self care. *Journal of Clinical Psychology, 58*(11), 1433-1441.

The Valley of Pursuing Nursing

This might be the deepest valley of all: the place where you begin to wonder if you were ever meant to be a nurse. Maybe you're lying in bed after a particularly difficult shift, questioning every career decision that led you to this point. Maybe you're looking at job postings in completely different fields and wondering if it's too late to start over. You might find yourself thinking: "Maybe I'm just not cut out for this. Maybe I made a mistake. Maybe I should have listened to the people who told me nursing would be too hard."

This valley is especially devastating because nursing often feels like more than a job—it feels like an identity. When you question whether you should be a nurse, you're questioning who you are at a fundamental level. But this valley teaches you the difference between loving the idea of nursing and finding your actual place within the profession. It forces you to examine what specifically isn't working and what changes might make nursing sustainable and fulfilling for you again.

When Valleys Signal System Problems

Not every valley is about personal growth. Sometimes valleys are warning signs that the system you're working in is broken, toxic, or unsustainable. Learning to distinguish between growth opportunities and system failures is essential for your wellbeing and career longevity.

If you're consistently experiencing moral distress because of inadequate staffing, that's not a valley that's teaching you resilience— that's a system problem that needs addressing. If your physical exhaustion stems from mandatory overtime and unsafe patient ratios, that's not building character—that's a workplace safety issue.

Signs that your valley might be system-related include:

- ➢ Problems that persist despite your best efforts to learn and grow
- ➢ Issues that affect all or most nurses in your workplace
- ➢ Situations where following hospital policy is impossible due to resource constraints
- ➢ Environments where reporting safety concerns leads to retaliation rather than improvement
- ➢ Workplaces where nurse wellbeing is consistently sacrificed for financial concerns

Recognizing system problems doesn't mean you're making excuses or lacking resilience. It means you're developing the professional wisdom to distinguish between challenges that will help you grow and situations that will simply wear you down.

Learning to Read Your Valleys

Not all valleys are created equal, and learning to read them correctly is a skill that develops with experience. Some valleys are temporary dips that come with normal learning and growth. Others are deeper depressions that signal the need for significant changes in your approach, your environment, or your career path. Temporary valleys often have clear triggers—a difficult patient death, a medication error, a conflict with a colleague. They're intense but relatively short-lived, and they typically resolve as you process the experience and integrate the lessons it offers.

Deeper valleys tend to be more persistent and pervasive. They affect multiple areas of your nursing practice and often extend into your personal life. They might signal the need for additional education, a change in specialty, or even a move to a different healthcare organization. The key is learning to sit with the discomfort of a valley long enough to understand what it's trying to teach you, while also recognizing when a valley is actually a sign that something needs to change.

When you're in a valley, especially a deep one, it can be tempting to make dramatic changes quickly. You might want to quit nursing entirely, transfer to a completely different unit, or make other major life decisions while you're in emotional distress.

But valleys teach patience as much as anything else. They teach you to sit with uncertainty, to gather information, and to make thoughtful decisions rather than reactive ones. Sometimes the path forward becomes clear only after you've spent enough time in the valley to fully understand what it's offering you. This doesn't mean you should accept every difficult situation as a growth opportunity. Physical or emotional abuse requires immediate action for your safety and wellbeing. But many valleys reward careful consideration and gradual response rather than hasty escape attempts.

Valleys aren't just about external complexity—they're about the internal battle, too. The hardest fight is often with yourself. It's the voice that says, "You're not enough." It's the whisper that suggests maybe you should have chosen a different path, that maybe you're not cut out for this after all.

When you find yourself in a valley, you're forced to pause, to look around, and to really see your surroundings for the first time. That internal voice telling you that you're not enough? It's not your enemy. It's actually trying to protect you, alerting you that something needs attention. The question isn't how to silence that voice, but how to listen to what it's really saying. Is it warning you about unsafe conditions that need addressing? Is it pushing you toward growth you've been avoiding? Is it highlighting skills you need to develop or boundaries you need to establish?

You've already won more battles than you give yourself credit for. The fact that you've made it this far means you have experience that no textbook could ever teach. You've developed instincts, wisdom, and resilience that are uniquely yours.

Your valleys aren't random detours—they're preparing you for something specific that only you can do. The maze isn't trying to trap you; it's shaping you into the nurse you're meant to be. Every valley you navigate brings you closer to finding not just any exit, but your unique path, the one that leads to where your unique purpose is. Each low point reveals another dimension of who you are as a nurse, another skill you didn't know you needed, another part of your unique purpose that can only be discovered at the bedside.

REFLECTION EXERCISE:

The Lessons of the Valley

You might surprise yourself with how much you've learned. Valleys may feel like defeat in the moment, but they often hold the keys to your greatest growth.

Take a moment to reflect on your hardest moment at the bedside:

- What did that experience teach you about your strength?
- How did you adapt in ways you didn't expect?
- What part of you grew because of that struggle?

CHAPTER FIVE

THE MINDSET RESET

Your Daily Escape Mechanism

Your thoughts can trap you faster than your hospital can.

In a well-known study from Stanford's Mind & Body Lab, psychologist Alia Crum explored how our beliefs shape the way our bodies respond to everyday work. She often shares the example of hotel housekeepers who were told that their daily tasks—vacuuming, scrubbing, lifting, bending—counted as exercise.

Nothing about their job changed. The only shift was how they thought about the work. Yet within a few weeks, these housekeepers showed measurable improvements: lower blood pressure, decreased body fat, and healthier body composition overall (Crum & Langer, 2007)[11]. Their mindset—not their workload—triggered the change.

---

[11] Crum, A. J., & Langer, E. J. (2007). *Mind-set matters: Exercise and the placebo effect.* Psychological Science, 18(2), 165–171. https://doi.org/10.1111/j.1467-9280.2007.01867.x

Crum explains that this effect isn't "wishful thinking" or vague positivity; it reflects how our beliefs shape our physiological and psychological responses. When we view an activity as beneficial, our bodies often respond in ways that support that belief (Crum & Langer, 2007)[12].

That insight raises a powerful question for nursing: If two nurses work identical shifts but one believes her challenges are strengthening her while the other sees them as slowly breaking her down, are they actually experiencing the same job?

Dr. Crum's research suggests they're not. The nurse who views her difficult patients, long hours, and stressful situations as building her resilience and expertise might literally have different stress hormone levels, better sleep, and more energy than the nurse who sees those same experiences as wearing her down. Their bodies and minds are responding to the same external events in completely different ways.

If your beliefs about your nursing challenges can actually change how your body responds to stress, how your brain processes problems, and how quickly you recover from difficult shifts, then isn't your mindset one of the most powerful tools in your nursing toolkit?

Rethinking the Maze: From Valleys to Doors

In the previous chapters, we explored how the valleys in your maze—those periods of feeling incompetent, experiencing moral distress, or questioning your calling—have been preparing you for something

[12] Crum, A. J., & Langer, E. J. (2007). *Mind-set matters: Exercise and the placebo effect.* Psychological Science, 18(2), 165–171. https://doi.org/10.1111/j.1467-9280.2007.01867.x

greater. As you emerge from those valleys with new wisdom and resilience, you're positioned to see your maze differently. The challenges that once felt demanding have taught you valuable lessons about yourself, about nursing, and about what you need to thrive at the bedside. This hard-won knowledge is exactly what allows you to spot opportunities that had been invisible before.

These opportunities have been there the whole time, doors hidden throughout the maze, tucked into your daily practice, disguised as routine tasks you've completed a thousand times. They look like regular parts of the maze—until you see them for what they really are: opportunities to fundamentally change your experience without changing your job. Most nurses never see these doors because they're moving too fast, too focused on survival.

Sometimes when we're under pressure, it feels like our only job is to survive the shift. We move faster. We push harder. We try to "fix" the feeling by doing more. But surviving and thriving are two very different things. If you only focus on escaping, you miss the real chances to change your experience right now—not months from now, but today, exactly where you are. What if I told you there are at least five doors around you right now? What if the professional experience you want isn't waiting for you on the other side of a resignation letter, but hidden within your current role, just a few steps in a different direction?

The Door of Mastery Over Motion

Most of us are praised for being fast, for multitasking, and doing more. You might find yourself rushing through assessments so you can "get ahead," only to realize you're missing important details in patient care that you used to catch easily. Research on cognitive load theory shows that when we try to process too many tasks simultaneously, our performance actually decreases rather than improves (Sweller, Ayres, & Kalyuga, 2011)[13]. Your brain isn't designed to multitask effectively, especially in high-stakes situations like healthcare.

Mastery over motion means shifting from frantic multitasking to intentional, focused action. It's choosing to move with clarity instead of speed, prioritizing what matters most rather than trying to do everything quickly so you can rush to the next task. When you operate from a place of mastery, even on your hardest days, you set the tone for how the shift flows.

This door is always open, but you won't find it while rushing. You find it when you slow down and become more intentional about the quality of your patient care.

Marcus's Story: From Surface to Depth

Marcus had been an ICU nurse for four years, priding himself on speed—getting bedside report done in under three minutes per patient, quickly scanning labs, and jumping straight into tasks. But his speed had become a liability, his rush through bedside reports created dangerous blind spots in his clinical picture. He had consistently missed the subtle

---

[13] Sweller, J., Ayres, P., & Kalyuga, S. (2011). *Cognitive Load Theory*. Springer. https://doi.org/10.1007/978-1-4419-8126-4

connections: the trending creatinine bump that had preceded the kidney failure, a family member's comment during report about the patient "acting different yesterday" that would have explained that day's delirium, and the correlation between the previous night's fluid imbalance and that morning's respiratory distress.

After his third patient crashed "unexpectedly" (the signs had been there), Marcus committed to mastery over one thing: data synthesis during report. Now he asks specific probing questions: "What was their baseline creatinine three days ago?" "When did that confusion actually start?" "How much did their weight change from admission?" He writes trends, not just numbers—drawing arrows, circling patterns, connecting yesterday's interventions to today's presentations.

This focused depth in a single area transformed his patient care: he now catches deterioration hours earlier, his questions during report have taught newer nurses what to watch for, and he hasn't been blindsided by a "sudden" change in months. Mastery wasn't about doing more—it was about going deeper into the data that was already there, waiting to be noticed.

By choosing depth over speed, Marcus finally found his door: it opened the moment he stopped rushing past the data and started listening to what it had been trying to tell him.

The Door of Strategic Relationships

The shift feels heavy when you believe you have to carry everything alone. Many nurses keep their heads down and just "handle it" because they don't want to be seen as needy or unprepared. Strategic relationships at the bedside can transform your entire work experience. The tech who consistently tells you when a patient looks different. The educator who sees your potential and offers guidance. The coworker who reminds you to take breaks and eat lunch. When you nurture these relationships, something shifts. These strategic relationships transform difficult shifts into manageable ones and good shifts into great ones. When others fail to open this door, the opportunities they miss become available to you. A new position perfectly suited to your skills might be shared with you before it's ever posted publicly.

You just have to start with one genuine conversation. One moment of openness. One offer to help when you're available. Your relationships aren't separate from your progression through the maze—they're connected to it.

Maria's Story: From Isolation to Connection

Maria was the PACU nurse who never asked for help. She would struggle alone to reposition a 300-pound post-op patient rather than appear needy to her colleagues. She skipped breaks instead of asking another nurse to cover her recovering patients. She troubleshot equipment problems herself, even when it took three times longer than asking someone who knew the fix.

She called it self-sufficiency. After two years, it had become exhausting. She was missing recovery cues she never would have missed before, and she had started dreading the drive to work.

Then one day, she asked Lisa, another PACU nurse, for help repositioning a patient. Lisa helped immediately—and then mentioned she had noticed some subtle color changes that Maria had missed while struggling on her own. Before they moved on, Lisa shared her method for catching early signs of respiratory depression.

That single conversation changed something in Maria.

She began taking an extra minute during OR handoff to ask the circulator real questions—about positioning challenges, unexpected blood loss, anything that might matter in recovery. She followed up with surgeons about specific post-op concerns. She checked in with floor nurses about how her patients did through the night.

Within months, her entire experience at work had transformed. OR nurses started offering details beyond the standard report—things like, "Watch her left arm, we had some trouble with positioning." Surgeons began stopping by to share patient-specific expectations for recovery. Floor nurses sent her updates that sharpened her clinical instincts in ways no continuing education course ever had.

The door to strategic relationships opened the moment Maria admitted she could not do everything alone. What she once feared would look like weakness became the foundation for the strongest work relationships she would ever have.

The Door of Self-Led Learning

Waiting for your hospital to hand you individualized professional growth is like waiting for your work email inbox to stop filling up. It's not going to happen. Individualized professional growth isn't something hospitals distribute. It's something you build by deciding to seek it out. Most healthcare organizations provide mandatory education focused on compliance and safety, but they rarely offer learning opportunities that address your specific interests or career goals. The learning that truly transforms your practice often comes from sources you choose yourself: a podcast about communication skills, an article about time management strategies, a conversation with a nurse from another specialty about how they handle difficult clinical situations.

Most nurses spend their careers in the passenger seat, allowing their nursing education department to chart their learning path. When you start choosing what you want to improve in your nursing practice instead of what someone else assigns, you take back the wheel and secure your position as the driver. Even ten minutes a week of intentional learning can reignite something exciting in you. The fact that you're reading this book right now means you've already opened this door. When you choose your own learning path, you're more engaged and more likely to apply what you learn. I actually have proof of this idea. In the book *The Adult Learner*, Knowles and his colleagues explain that adults learn best when they have control over their own growth (Knowles et al., 2015)[14]. They show how self-directed learning leads to deeper engagement, stronger motivation, and more meaningful retention because adults choose what matters to them—instead of passively completing mandatory training.

---

[14] Knowles, M. S., Holton III, E. F., & Swanson, R. A. (2015). The adult learner: The definitive classic in adult education and human resource development (8th ed.). Routledge.

Derek's Story: From Passive to Intentional

Derek completed every mandatory education module his hospital required. Annual competencies, safety protocols, new EMR training— he did it all. He pretty much just checked his nursing education boxes. He never pushed himself to learn beyond what was assigned.

After five years on his medical-surgical floor, he could manage five patients efficiently. He was competent. But he also felt trapped. He found himself increasingly frustrated by the diabetic patients who kept getting readmitted, and he could not explain why certain wound care instructions worked better than others. He knew there were gaps in his knowledge. He just kept waiting for someone else to fill them.

Then he decided to stop waiting.

He started small. After his first shift each week, he listened to a fifteen-minute podcast about patient education techniques on his drive home. One episode mentioned a free online course on motivational interviewing for medication compliance, so he enrolled. He started picking the wound care nurses' brains about diabetic wound management. He also purchased an e-book on discharge planning. But his real education came from a journal he kept where he collected patient feedback on what made diabetic education so difficult to follow—insights no textbook could have given him.

Within six months, Derek's discharge teaching had become the template that other nurses copied. His manager noticed him showing newer nurses the engagement techniques he had picked up from his podcast and invited him to lead a unit-based project on patient education effectiveness. This was an opportunity that never would have been offered to him before. The project's success got him noticed beyond his unit. The Director of Infection Prevention invited him to collaborate on a hospital-wide initiative—and what started as a single meeting became an ongoing mentorship that opened doors Derek never knew were there.

The door to self-led learning opened the moment Derek stopped relying on annual competencies to make his care meaningful—and started teaching himself what his patients actually needed.

The Door of Controlled Contribution

You can't fix everything wrong with healthcare, but you can contribute something meaningful within your sphere of influence. The difference between feeling helpless and feeling hopeful often comes down to one decision—choosing where to focus your energy. You might decide to become the nurse known for giving exceptional reports, the kind that help the oncoming shift start with confidence instead of confusion. Or you might focus on being the calming presence when a code is called and everyone else is rattled. Or maybe your thing becomes discharging patients home—making sure your patients actually understand what comes next so the car ride home feels less overwhelming.

This door isn't about doing more tasks or taking on additional responsibilities. It's about identifying one area where your unique skills and perspective can make a difference and committing to excellence in that space. This door is about job crafting. Job crafting is the practice of reshaping your role through small, intentional moves rather than waiting for someone else to fix what is not working (Wrzesniewski & Dutton, 2001)[15]. The nurses who do this do not have easier assignments or better ratios. They simply stop treating their job like something that happens to them and start treating it like something they have a hand in creating.

James's Story: How One Nurse Changed What Gets Shared

James was a cardiac step-down nurse who made the same phone calls every shift. He would update families with clinical facts—and they would listen politely. Then they would ask the same questions again, still confused, still scared. Nothing he said seemed to land.

And in their hospital beds, the patients carried worries they never put into words. Everyone was afraid, and no one was connecting.

James watched this pattern for months, and it wore on him. He could not prevent heart attacks. He could not guarantee outcomes. He could not control when anyone got discharged. So he let it keep happening, night after night, because he did not know what else to do.

Then one shift, he decided to try something different. He would bridge the gap that everyone else had simply accepted.

---

[15] Wrzesniewski, A., & Dutton, J. E. (2001). Crafting a job: Revisioning employees as active crafters of their work. *Academy of Management Review, 26*(2), 179-201. https://doi.org/10.5465/amr.2001.4378011

He started being more intentional about something he was already doing—calling families with updates. But instead of leading with clinical facts alone, he added something else. Before the end of each shift, he spent a few extra minutes with his patients. He asked about their day. He noticed the small victories and asked about them directly. "You walked to the bathroom this morning without much help. How did that feel? What are you thinking about now?" His patients would open up. They would tell him what they were looking forward to—sitting on the porch, getting home to their cats, working in the garden again. James wrote it all down.

When he called families that evening, he combined progress with forward thinking. "Your dad had a really good day. He walked to the bathroom on his own and felt confident about it. He is already thinking about getting home and sitting on the porch with you. When you call him tonight, ask him how that walk felt. Talk about what comes next."

Families started calling their loved ones with specific things to talk about—how the walk went, what the doctor said about moving to another floor, whether the new medication was helping. They were no longer dealing with the fear of hospitalization in isolation. They were tracking recovery together. They had real conversations instead of anxious silence.

One daughter wrote to the unit manager: "James gave me updates that were thoughtful and timely. We stopped dreading my father's calls and started looking forward to them. We are on the same page again."

The door to controlled contribution opened the moment James admitted what he could actually influence. Not outcomes. Not policy. He did not cure heart disease or take on extra responsibilities. He simply decided that one thing—bridging the gap between frightened patients and helpless families—would be done with excellence and intention.

The Door of Identity Beyond the Role

One of the most insidious effects of long shifts is how they make you forget who you are outside the hospital. You stop seeing yourself as a whole person and start defining yourself by your last shift, your patient satisfaction scores, your flawless performance review, or the biggest mistake you made in front of your peers. But you are so much more than your nursing role.

Nursing can consume your identity without you even realizing it's happening. You start thinking of yourself primarily as a nurse, and everything else becomes secondary. Your hobbies disappear. Your non-healthcare friendships fade. Your interests outside of work seem less important.

Reclaiming your identity beyond nursing means remembering the parts of you that existed before the badge: your creativity, your sense of humor, your curiosity about the world, your dreams that have nothing to do with patient ratios or charting audits. When you nurture these aspects of yourself, you often find renewed energy for your nursing role as well. You can't pour from an empty cup, and maintaining your full humanity actually makes you a better nurse.

Rachel's Story: Reclaiming the Person Behind the Badge

Rachel had been a nurse for eight years, and somewhere along the way, she'd stopped being anything else. She used to play guitar—not professionally, just for herself, late at night when the world was quiet. She had friends outside healthcare who actually knew her. She read novels. She took photographs on weekend hikes. But over time, those things got crowded out. Night shifts made hobbies seem frivolous. The emotional weight of work made socializing feel exhausting. Her identity slowly narrowed until she could only describe herself in relation to her job: "I'm a critical care nurse. I work at the hospital."

The breaking point came when her old college friend asked what she'd been doing lately. Rachel opened her mouth to answer and realized every single thing she was about to say involved the hospital. There was nothing else. When she hung up the phone, she felt the weight of it: she had become only her job.

So Rachel started small. She took her guitar out of the closet—dusty, slightly out of tune—and played one song. The next week she played two songs. This same week she texted her non-nursing friend and made plans for coffee. She picked up a novel and read actual chapters instead of scrolling through her phone. She later signed up for a run-walk event in the park close to her apartment.

Within months, something shifted. Rachel was still working at the bedside in critical care. But when she clocked out, she was someone other than a nurse. She was a person who played guitar badly but looked forward to the moment.

She was a friend who actually showed up. She was curious about the world again. And strangely, this made her better at her job. She had energy she didn't know she'd lost. She had perspective. She had something to look forward to besides her next shift.

Her coworkers noticed. She laughed more. When a patient was having a hard day, Rachel didn't just move through the motions—she brought actual presence, because she had something left to give.

One night a patient asked her what she did for fun, and instead of dodging the question with "Oh, just sleep between shifts," she said, "I play guitar, actually." The patient smiled. They talked about music for ten minutes. Can you imagine working at the bedside and not having any of these small but meaningful moments? I would say that without these moments a nurse may feel trapped in their bedside role.

Rachel discovered that the door to identity beyond her role opened the moment she admitted that nursing wasn't enough to define her— it was better when it was one part of a whole life.

She didn't have to choose between being a good nurse and having a life. In fact, rediscovering her old self made her a better nurse. Her hospital badge still mattered. But it was no longer all she was.

Open One Door at a Time

None of this is easy. I want to be honest with you about that.

Maria had to swallow her pride and ask for help when everything in her screamed to handle it alone. Derek had to admit that checking boxes was not the same as growing. James had to accept that he could not fix what was broken. Each of them stood at a door they were not sure they wanted to open. They pushed through anyway. That is what this chapter is really about. Not five magic doors that make bedside nursing suddenly painless. There is no such thing. The work may still be hard. There will still be shifts that take more than you have to give. But there is a difference between hard and hopeless. The difference is your decision.

You create solid ground when you master one thing instead of drowning in everything. You stop carrying the weight alone when you build real relationships with the people around you. You find breathing room when you focus your energy on what you can actually shape and release what you cannot. You have something left to give when you protect who you are outside these walls. And you stop letting the bad days define you. You can now see and confidently explain the five doors. None of them require permission. None of them require a better unit or a more supportive manager. They only require you as you are right now. Tired. Frustrated. Not sure any of this will work. That version of you is enough to open the first door. Open one and see what happens. Then open another.

YOUR UNIQUE PERSPECTIVE

CHAPTER SIX

THE KEY TO BREAKING OUT

Your Unique Purpose Within Bedside Nursing

A nurse without a purpose is a nurse at risk for burnout.

There's a story about an adult elephant, powerful enough to topple trees, who routinely stands motionless in the middle of a circus tent. As a calf, a thin rope around its ankle convinced the elephant that movement was impossible. Years passed. The rope was removed but the elephant never tested whether it could break free. The memory of being held became stronger than the physical restraint ever was. If you aren't careful, you'll become that elephant. Standing in the middle of your unit, surrounded by endless tasks. Believing you're stuck exactly where you are. And the circus? It's counting on you never testing that rope.

That elephant may have a great memory, but it doesn't understand its purpose. This chapter will help you rediscover the deep reason behind why you care, why you show up, and why your work matters. That elephant will likely stay in the circus for life. But you? You've come this far, which means you're not the same nurse who started this book.

You are actively moving through your maze without any ropes attached. Those doors that were invisible? They are now easier to notice. And those bedside skills you've been dismissing as "just being a nurse"? You now know they are the foundation for something bigger. Everything you've discovered in this book so far has been preparing you for your unique purpose within bedside nursing.

You've proven you can break free. But real freedom isn't just about having options—it's about knowing which door is yours. That's what your unique know-how reveals.

What Is Your Unique Know-How?

What if I told you there's another door? Not one that pulls you away from bedside nursing, but one that takes you deeper into what you're actually building at the bedside. Your unique know-how lives where three things meet, and I guarantee you've been underestimating at least one of them.

> **Your Skill:** The clinical and interpersonal abilities that set you apart from the crowd. These are the skills you trust when you want to perform at your best.

> **Your Passion:** The parts of nursing that still matter to you, the specific work that energizes rather than drains you.

> ➤ **Your Perspective:** This is shaped by every life experience you've ever had. No one else sees nursing through your eyes, and that's not a weakness. *This is your unique strength.*

Together, these create the conditions for peak experiences—when a challenge meets both your skill and your passion, you get to leverage your unique perspective, and slip effortlessly into the flow of your best work.

Your unique know-how isn't just another door in the maze—it's the key. You can't open the right doors until you know what key you're holding. Throughout this book, you've been developing the ability to see patterns, recognize new doors, and identify new paths forward. Now, let's discuss the steps to uncovering your unique purpose.

The Five-Step Process to Uncover Your Unique Purpose

Step 1: Identify Your Skill

Think back over the last month—the actual month you lived through and answer this honestly:

What do your colleagues consistently ask you for help with? Every nurse on your unit has that one thing. Maybe they come to you when they need to have a difficult conversation with a family. Maybe they ask you to take the most challenging patient assignments. Maybe they seek you out when they need someone to mentor the new grad who's about to quit. This pattern isn't random. It's your colleagues recognizing something in you that you might not even see yourself.

The skill you want to be known for might be different from the one you're already known for, and that's perfectly fine. But you should start with what's true right now, and work on the skills you hope to master someday.

Step 2: Explore Your Professional Passions

What part of nursing consistently energizes you rather than drains you? What makes you forget you're supposed to be tired?

Most nurses think they should be passionate about the noble parts of nursing—the life-saving moments, the grateful families, the meaningful connections. But maybe what energizes you is the intellectual puzzle of figuring out why the patient in room 312 keeps having syncopal episodes that no one can explain. Maybe you love the dynamic complexity of a trauma bay, or the quiet satisfaction of getting all the confused patients to take their medications without a fight. Maybe you're energized by teaching the new nurses how to chart efficiently, or by advocating for policy changes that actually complement your unit's workflow. This energy source isn't just about job satisfaction—it's your internal compass pointing toward your unique purpose.

Step 3: Own Your Perspective

Your perspective is shaped by everything you've lived through, and that includes the hard stuff. Maybe you've been on the other side of the bed rail as a patient or a caregiver. Maybe you've seen what happens when healthcare fails someone you love. Maybe you grew up in a family that didn't trust doctors, or maybe you're the first person in your family to work in healthcare at all. These experiences sharpen your ability to notice details that escape other nurses. Your perspective isn't just part of your story—it's the lens through which you discover your unique purpose within nursing.

Think about it: if you've personally experienced what it's like to feel afraid in a hospital, you might naturally gravitate toward comforting anxious patients. If you've watched a family member struggle with complex medical instructions, you might find yourself drawn to patient education. If you've seen how small acts of kindness can make an impossible day bearable, you might become the nurse who specializes in making people feel seen and heard.

Your perspective is a powerful advantage that's directing you toward your unique way of serving patients.

Step 4: Find Your People

Once you find out what makes you different, it's time to find people who get it. Not people who tolerate your interests, but people who share them and see their value. This community might exist within your current workplace, but it probably extends far beyond it. If you're passionate about wound care, join the Wound, Ostomy, and Continence Nurses Society. If you love emergency nursing, connect with your local and national Emergency Nurses Association officers. If you're all about patient education, find groups focused on health literacy.

Don't just join—participate. Share what you know. Ask questions. Be the person who shows up. Because when you find your community, you're not just networking. You're discovering how your unique purpose fits into something bigger than yourself. Your community can bring credibility to your purpose and professional mission. These colleagues serve as your professional advocates, understanding your unique perspective and contributions in ways that transcend typical professional relationships.

Step 5: Build Your Personal Brand Around Your Know-How

Your personal brand isn't about becoming a social media influencer. It's about being intentional about how you show up and what you want to be known for. It's about making your unique know-how visible so that the right opportunities, people, and situations can find you.

- ➤ **Define your know-how in one sentence**: What specific problem can you uniquely solve? What value do you bring to the bedside that others don't?

- ➤ **Share your knowledge consistently**: This could be as simple as being the nurse who always has the latest evidence-based practice information or as complex as writing articles for nursing journals.

- ➤ **Collaborate strategically**: Look for projects, committees, or initiatives that align with your unique know-how and allow you to express it.

Your goal isn't self-promotion. It's alignment. When you're clear about your purpose, other people can be clear about it too.

Here's what I've learned: Inside the maze, your current skills can help you navigate your circumstances more effectively. Your passions guide you toward the path meant for you—not anyone else. And your perspective gives you the language to express what makes you different from every other nurse out there. Master these three, and you've begun the journey toward discovering your unique purpose.

Discovering your unique know-how moves you forward with newfound clarity, transforming what once felt like an overwhelming maze into your own distinct path—one where even the toughest days work to your advantage. But I need to be honest with you about something important. If you do this work and realize that your purpose genuinely lies outside of bedside nursing, that path is just as legitimate and worthy of action. After discovering your unique skills, passions, and perspective, pay close attention to what energizes you— if that activity doesn't happen at the bedside, that's not a problem the bedside will fix. Leaving bedside nursing because your purpose lies elsewhere isn't a bad move; it's a courageous act of honoring what you've discovered about yourself. So if that's your truth, here's the one action I'd recommend: take everything you've discovered about your skills, passions, and perspective, and write out how these translate into value for the role that you think would be a better fit for you away from the bedside.

I believe when you're connected to your unique purpose, you're more resilient against the problems that cause others to professionally burn out. That resilience becomes your unique advantage when paired with strategic problem-solving. You'll have this advantage in whatever role you pursue once you've found your unique purpose. In the next chapter, we'll discuss how to strategically think your way out of feeling trapped. Finding your unique path to your unique purpose should be your ultimate professional goal, and my goal is to help you get there.

CHAPTER SEVEN

STRATEGIC THINKING FOR TRAPPED NURSES

Problem-Solving Your Way Out

Feeling trapped is often a thinking problem before it's a career problem.

want you to picture something. You climb and lift your head above the walls of your current circumstances. You see a part of the maze you didn't know existed. You notice a new route. You spot a weakness in the system. You find a solution no one else saw because they never stopped long enough to look up.

That's what real problem-solving feels like. It starts with one bold moment of clarity. When you give yourself permission to pause and look at the bigger picture, you begin to notice where things could be better. You start identifying patterns, waste, inefficiencies, or daily frustrations that could become stepping stones toward real change.

But here's a crucial fact to understand: not every problem deserves your obsession.

Some frustrations are better left alone. Some are distractions. Some are systemic and very hard to change. Others are clues pointing you toward work that matters deeply to you. Some problems are highly visible but have minimal impact on what really matters. Others might be less obvious but represent significant opportunities for improvement. The "right" problem is one that intersects your unique know-how with a genuine need that, when solved, creates value your leaders can recognize and measure.

So how do you know which problems are worth your time, energy, and focus?

Start by listening to your emotional cues, but filter them through a strategic lens. According to Susan David's research on emotional agility, emotions like irritation and disappointment are not problems to ignore—they are signals that something matters to you (David, 2016)[16]. When something consistently frustrates you, it's often because it conflicts with a core value that matters deeply to you as a nurse. But the key is asking yourself: does this frustration point to something that also matters to my manager, my patients, or the organization's bottom line?

Ask yourself: When do I feel most frustrated? When do I catch myself saying, "It shouldn't have to be this way"? Then follow up with the

---

[16] David, S. (2016). *Emotional agility: Get unstuck, embrace change, and thrive in work and life.* Avery.

strategic questions: Who else is affected by this problem? What measurable outcomes could improve if this were solved? These questions shift your mindset from general complaints to targeted problem-solving, helping you engage with issues that capture the attention of those who can open new pathways away from the bedside.

You can also scan your shift for friction points that have broader implications. Friction is anything that slows down good care, wastes time, or drains energy. These may not be the problems you can solve immediately, but they help you build awareness of where small, meaningful changes can create ripple effects throughout your healthcare system.

When you find a problem that connects to your values and aligns with organizational goals, you unlock motivation that no paycheck can match. You don't need to solve everything. You just need to name one thing that matters deeply to you and to the people who have the power to implement change.

Discover the Real Problem, Not the Obvious One

Here are five powerful techniques that can help you not only solve problems on your floor but also discover new avenues for growth and engagement, both in and outside of direct patient care.

1. Begin with the End in Mind: Picture the Goal and Work Backward

In *The 7 Habits of Highly Effective People*, Stephen Covey teaches that the most effective people start by picturing their ideal outcome and then work backward to guide their decisions—a principle he calls 'Begin With the End in Mind' (Covey, 1989)[17]. When you feel trapped at the bedside, this principle works in reverse: instead of starting with your current frustration and trying to solve your way out, you picture yourself *not* feeling trapped anymore—and work backward to discover what's actually missing right now.

How It Works for Nurses: Picture the version of yourself who feels fully engaged, valued, and purposeful at the bedside—what does that look like? Maybe you're influencing unit-level decisions, or your clinical insights are shaping policy, or you're mentoring newer nurses in ways that matter. Now work backward: What would need to be true for that version of you to exist? Perhaps leaders would need to see evidence of your strategic thinking. What would need to happen before that? You'd need documented examples of problems you've identified and solutions you've proposed. What comes before that? You'd need to start capturing your observations instead of letting them disappear shift after shift. Suddenly, you've reverse-engineered the trapped feeling: you're not trapped by bedside nursing itself— you're trapped by invisibility, by insights that die in your head because they're never written down.

Why It Works: This method works because most nurses who feel trapped can't articulate what "not trapped" would actually look like— they just know they want out. When you envision your ideal state and

---

[17] Covey, S. R. (1989). *The 7 habits of highly effective people: Powerful lessons in personal change.* Free Press.

trace backward, you discover the specific conditions that are missing: autonomy, influence, intellectual challenge, recognition, purpose beyond tasks. That clarity transforms "I need to escape bedside nursing" into "I need three specific things to change for me to thrive here"—and those are problems you can solve without abandoning the clinical work you're actually good at. *The trapped feeling loses its grip once you see exactly what freedom would require.*

2. First Principles Thinking: Get to the Root of What You Really Want

Richard Feynman's problem-solving approach exemplified "First Principles Thinking": he would strip away conventional assumptions to identify the fundamental truths underlying a problem, then rebuild understanding from those core elements. This approach encourages breaking things down to their most basic components before building solutions from the ground up (Feynman, 1985)[18]. When you feel trapped at the bedside, you're often trapped not by reality but by assumptions you've inherited—"bedside nurses don't influence policy," "you have to leave the floor to have impact," "clinical work means you can't be a leader." First Principles Thinking dismantles those inherited beliefs and asks: what's actually true?

How It Works for Nurses: Instead of accepting "I feel trapped at the bedside" as a one-sided truth, break it down to the irreducible elements. Ask: What specifically makes me feel trapped? Strip away the assumptions.

---

[18] Feynman, R. P. (1985). *Surely you're joking, Mr. Feynman!: Adventures of a curious character.* W. W. Norton & Company.

"I can't make a difference here"—is that fundamentally true, or is it that you haven't documented your ideas in ways leaders can act on?

Why It Works: First Principles Thinking works because that trapped feeling isn't built on facts—it's built on assumptions you've never questioned. When you strip away everything you've been told about bedside nursing and examine only what's provably true, "I'm trapped at the bedside" often becomes "I feel trapped when no one sees what I contribute." That's not a career crisis—that's a visibility problem. And visibility problems have solutions. By questioning every assumption about what bedside work has to mean, you stop treating the walls around you as permanent and start testing them. Some walls are real. But most? *They're just beliefs you inherited from burned-out coworkers and outdated systems. Once you see which is which, you realize you were never as trapped as you thought.*

3. The Five Whys: Dig Deeper to Find the True Opportunity

The Five Whys technique, developed by Sakichi Toyoda in the 1930s at Toyota Industries, involves asking 'why' five times to uncover the root cause of a problem. The method became a cornerstone of the Toyota Production System under Taiichi Ohno's leadership, proving that most problems have layers—and the first answer you get is rarely the whole truth (Ohno, 1988)[19]. When you feel trapped at the bedside, your initial explanation is usually just the surface symptom, not the actual source of your dissatisfaction.

---

[19] Ohno, T. (1988). *Toyota production system: Beyond large-scale production.* Productivity Press.

How It Works for Nurses: Start with the feeling: "Why do I feel trapped at the bedside?" Your first answer might be, "Because I'm exhausted." Ask why again: "Why am I exhausted?" Perhaps it's "Because the work feels repetitive." Why does repetitive work exhaust you? "Because I'm not using my brain the way I want to." Why does that matter? "Because I have insights about how things could improve, but no one listens." Why does no one listen? "Because I haven't documented what I see in a way they can act on." Suddenly, you've moved from "I'm trapped and exhausted" to "I have valuable insights but lack the communication structure to make them visible." That's a completely different—and solvable—problem.

Why It Works: The Five Whys works because that trapped feeling is almost never what you think it is on day one. You might believe you're trapped by the physical demands, the schedule, or the patients—but five layers down, you discover you're actually trapped by invisibility, by knowing you could contribute at a higher level but not knowing how to make that contribution count. Each "why" peels back another layer of the real issue, and by the fifth one, you're face-to-face with the actual barrier between you and feeling valued, engaged, and purposeful at the bedside. *Once you see the real problem, you stop trying to escape nursing entirely and start solving the specific thing that's actually in your way.*

4. The 80/20 Principle (Pareto Principle): Focus on High-Impact Skills

When you feel trapped at the bedside, it's rarely because *everything* is wrong—it's usually because a vital few sources of frustration are creating a disproportionate amount of your dissatisfaction. The Pareto Principle, originally observed by economist Vilfredo Pareto in 1896 when he noted that 80% of Italy's wealth was held by 20% of the population, was later generalized by quality management pioneer Joseph M. Juran. Applied to your career, this principle suggests that approximately 20% of your daily experiences are generating 80% of that trapped feeling you can't shake (Pareto, 1896[20]; Juran, 1951)[21].

How It Works for Nurses: Instead of accepting that "bedside nursing just feels like this," use the 80/20 lens to identify the specific few factors causing most of your dissatisfaction. Is it the lack of autonomy in decision-making? The repetitive nature of certain tasks that don't utilize your critical thinking? Feeling invisible despite your expertise? The physical toll without intellectual challenge? When you pinpoint the vital few sources—perhaps it's just 2-3 specific aspects of bedside work—you can address those strategically rather than feeling overwhelmed by the entirety of your role.

Why It Works: The 80/20 Principle works because that trapped feeling isn't actually about everything at the bedside—it's about specific, identifiable conditions that, once named, lose their power to paralyze you. When you discover that 80% of your frustration comes from, say, lack of influence over unit decisions, feeling like your clinical judgment doesn't matter beyond the shift, and missing intellectual challenge, suddenly you're not trapped by "bedside

---

[20] Pareto, V. (1896). *Cours d'économie politique professé à l'Université de Lausanne.* Lausanne: F. Rouge.
[21] *Juran, J. M. (1951). Quality control handbook. McGraw-Hill.*

nursing"—you're facing three solvable problems. You can stay at the bedside and address those three things (document your insights, propose solutions, seek projects that challenge you strategically) without needing to abandon clinical care entirely. *The clarity transforms "I'm trapped and have to leave" into "I need to change these specific conditions"—and that's a problem you can actually solve.*

5. SWOT Analysis: Objectively Assess Opportunities and Threats

SWOT analysis (Strengths, Weaknesses, Opportunities, Threats), developed by Albert Humphrey and colleagues at the Stanford Research Institute during the 1960s-1970s, is a structured framework for evaluating a situation objectively while considering strategic implications (Humphrey, 2005)[22]. When you feel trapped at the bedside, this framework stops you from spiraling in vague dissatisfaction and forces you to inventory the actual landscape you're standing in—what you have working for you, what's legitimately holding you back, what doors are actually open, and what barriers are real versus imagined.

Here's a SWOT analysis example:

> ➢ *Strengths:* What do you bring that others don't?

> ➢ *Weaknesses:* What's legitimately missing that contributes to your trapped feeling?

---

[22] Humphrey, A. (2005). SWOT analysis for management consulting. *SRI Alumni Newsletter (TOWS matrix).*

> ➤ *Opportunities:* What pathways exist right now that you haven't noticed?

> ➤ *Threats:* What's genuinely blocking progress versus what you're assuming?

Why It Works: SWOT analysis works because the trapped feeling thrives on ambiguity—when everything feels wrong, nothing feels fixable. This framework forces brutal clarity: you discover you have more strengths than you're leveraging (your clinical judgment, your frontline perspective, your relationships), your weaknesses are specific and learnable (not character flaws), the opportunities are more available than you realized (committees, pilot programs, informal influence), and some threats are real barriers while others are just stories you're telling yourself. Once you see the actual map—what you truly have, what you actually need, what's genuinely possible, and what's legitimately hard—the trapped feeling shifts from "I'm powerless" to "I'm standing in specific terrain with specific options." That's the difference between feeling stuck in a maze and recognizing you're just at a crossroads that requires a strategic choice.

It's a great idea to prioritize opportunities that match your organization's strategic goals—especially areas where your unique strengths can neutralize real threats to patient outcomes and operational efficiency.

When you feel trapped in the routine of bedside nursing, it can be hard to believe there's a way forward that doesn't involve leaving the bedside entirely. But often, what feels like an obstacle is actually a moment asking for a new perspective. The problems that frustrate you most might be the exact places where you can lead. These five strategies are not quick fixes, but they can help you step back and see the possibilities in front of you. Your frustration isn't a sign you're in the wrong place—it's a signal that you're ready to lead from where you stand.

REFLECTION ACTIVITY:
Choose Your Problem-Solving Approach

Stop here and reflect on the questions below:

- Which technique resonates with you the most? Why?
- What's one problem you'd like to approach differently? How could using this new approach help you see the situation from a new perspective?
- What's the first step you'll take to apply this technique in your daily work or career planning?

CHAPTER EIGHT

THE ULTIMATE ADVANTAGE

The Hidden Power Every Bedside Nurse Already Possesses

If it's not documented, it's not done.
– Common Healthcare Documentation Standard

There's a skill that separates ordinary bedside nurses from those who become influential leaders and change makers. It's not another certification or a clinical technique that requires years to master. This powerful ability has been waiting patiently in your hands all along, ready to elevate you to a class entirely your own.

Let's step into this scene: You've just peeled off your scrubs after a twelve-hour shift. You're sitting in your favorite chair, legs finally resting, replaying the day's events. These events are profound human experiences wrapped in doctor's orders and your facility's documentation requirements. Yet these powerful stories often disappear into the ether, lost in the flurry of charting and checklists, buried under the weight of your next shift. What if you captured not just the dramatic saves and the medical miracles, but also the quiet victories?

You already possess experiences that could reshape the maze of bedside nursing. You've navigated impossible situations with grace, advocated for patients who had no voice, and found solutions that textbooks never taught you. The gap between experiencing something powerful and creating lasting change from it comes down to one critical skill—a skill so fundamental that it's often overlooked, yet so transformative that it separates those who remain trapped in their circumstances from those who rise above them.

This skill turns your personal memories into messages that travel beyond your unit, your hospital, your city and state. It doesn't just document reality; it has the power to create a new professional path.

It becomes your tool for reflection, helping you extract wisdom from complexity. This skill becomes your bridge to inspiration, connecting your individual struggles to universal truths that resonate with others. Most importantly, it connects the often invisible emotional labor you perform every day with the larger conversation about what nursing is and what it could be.

When you master this skill, you don't just set yourself apart as another good nurse. You become a leader whose voice carries weight far beyond your immediate surroundings.

That skill is writing.

Why Being Great Isn't Good Enough

Being exceptional at your job isn't enough anymore. I want you to consider this skill that complements all that you have learned in this book and throughout your career. My goal isn't to convince you to be a novelist. My goal is to help you move from feeling trapped to discovering new opportunities at the bedside, and for many nurses, consistent writing can help open new doors. The nurses who rise above their circumstances, who influence change and shape conversations, understand something crucial: doing great work in silence is like being the most talented musician in the world but never performing for an audience. We all need a method of sharing our exceptional thoughts with the world. Think about the nurses whose voices you recognize and respect. They didn't become influential by keeping their insights to themselves. They found ways to share what they learned, what they observed, what they discovered in the trenches of healthcare. It's very difficult to share what you can't remember. I've discovered that writing, journaling, or just making notes are great ways to hold onto your own thinking. Your experiences are uniquely yours, but the lessons they contain are universally valuable.

Writing gives you the stage to perform in front of your audience. This one skill transforms your insights from private thoughts into public contributions. Whether you start with a private journal that nobody else ever sees or eventually share your perspectives through professional blogs, social media, or even formal publications, writing positions you as someone whose perspective matters. When you write about the patient who taught you something profound about suffering, or the family who showed you a new way to think about grief, or the colleague who demonstrated what real teamwork looks like, you're offering gifts that other nurses desperately need. Your written thoughts can spark conversations in break rooms, influence policy discussions, and change how people think about patient care.

In the last chapter you were encouraged to think strategically—writing is a tool that captures that thinking and turns it into career-changing leverage. Success in any field rarely happens in isolation. Nursing presents a unique challenge: we're scattered across shifts, units, hospitals, and cities. We might work side by side with the same people for years but never really know their stories, their struggles, their insights. Writing changes that dynamic completely. If you ever decide to share your writing with the public, you have an opportunity to reach nurses you've never met who are fighting similar battles, celebrating similar victories, learning similar lessons.

Imagine a nurse in Seattle reading about your experience with a difficult patient and thinking, "Finally, someone who gets it." Picture a new graduate in Miami finding courage in your story about making a critical mistake and learning from it. Envision a seasoned nurse in rural Montana feeling less alone because your words perfectly captured something she's felt but never been able to express. Your authenticity becomes a magnet that draws like-minded people into your orbit. You stop being just another nurse going through the motions and become someone other nurses want to know, learn from, and work alongside.

The conversations that grow from your writing can lead to mentorships, collaborative projects, speaking opportunities, and career paths you never imagined. These connections can create a new path in the maze.

Creating a Legacy That Outlasts Your Career

Think about the nurses who influenced you most during your career. What do you remember about them? Chances are, it's not just their clinical skills or their efficiency with tasks. It's the wisdom they shared, the perspectives they offered, the way they helped you see situations differently. Now imagine if those insights had been written down. Picture having access to their thoughts about difficult cases, their reflections on what they learned from decades of practice, their advice for navigating the challenges you're facing now. Writing creates that legacy for the nurses who come after you. Every reflection you capture, every lesson you document, every story you tell becomes part of a larger narrative about what it means to be a nurse in this era of healthcare. Your experiences matter not just to you, but to the nursing student who will read your words five years from now and think, "I'm not alone in feeling this way." They matter to the policy makers who need to understand the real human impact of their decisions.

If you've never thought of yourself as a writer, that's not what this is about. Capturing your bedside stories in whatever form—rough notes, fragments, honest reflections—is a skill that develops with practice, and honestly, it's one you should consider. Years from now, when you've moved into different roles or perhaps retired entirely, your written reflections can continue to influence, inspire, and guide others. Your voice can still be part of the conversation, still contributing to the profession's growth and evolution.

Your experiences contain solutions because they emerge from the front lines. Your stories have power because they bridge the gap between what healthcare claims to be and what it actually is. The hidden power you already possess isn't waiting to be discovered—it's waiting to be unleashed. From exactly where you're sitting right now, with the experiences you've already lived and the insights you've already gained. Through writing, you discover that your unique purpose isn't something separate from bedside nursing—it can be revealed within it, one story at a time.

This is one of your ultimate advantages.

REFLECTION ACTIVITY:
Your First Story

Take a few minutes to write about one meaningful moment. Reflect on the following:

- What happened, and how did it make you feel?
- What did you learn from that moment?
- How might your story help someone else understand the importance of nursing?

CHAPTER NINE

THE IMPACT OF MEETING THE RIGHT PERSON

A Connection that Can Change Your Path

The strongest bridges are built long before you need to cross them.

Imagine yourself three hours into what feels like an impossible shift when you watch a seasoned nurse glide through a crisis that would have sent you spiraling. Their composure, clinical judgment, and natural leadership seem almost effortless. What looks like natural talent is actually the accumulated wisdom of countless colleagues, mentors, and peers who invested in that nurse's growth along the way.

This moment illustrates a fundamental truth about nursing: professional growth in the maze isn't a solo journey, no matter what we tell ourselves during those long, isolating shifts. Our journey is deeply integrated with the connections we build and the relationships that challenge us to see beyond our current circumstances.

The right person at the right time can change everything about your career. But not every professional relationship becomes transformative. The ones that do share specific characteristics that set them apart. They serve different purposes at different times— offering shelter during a crisis, pushing you toward growth you didn't think you were ready for, or opening doors you didn't even know existed. The most powerful careers aren't built in isolation; they're built in the presence of people who see your potential more clearly than you see it yourself.

The question isn't whether you need these connections. You do. The real question is: what exactly makes a connection career-changing? What are the specific qualities and roles that separate meaningful professional relationships from the polite, surface-level interactions that fill most of our workdays? Understanding this matters because once you know what to look for—and what to offer—you can be intentional about building the kind of network that actually changes your trajectory.

Not every professional relationship becomes transformative, but the ones that do share specific characteristics that set them apart. These are the connections that fundamentally alter how you see yourself and your possibilities. The bedside shapes you, but certain people help you recognize what that shaping has actually created.

The Authentic Supporter

True professional supporters don't just offer advice; they create safe spaces for vulnerability and growth. They're the ones who check in after your difficult shifts, celebrate your small wins, and remind you of your strengths when burnout has you questioning everything. This support becomes exponentially more powerful when it comes from someone who genuinely invests in your success—someone who listens without judgment, validates your experiences, and helps you process challenges in ways that promote growth rather than resignation.

Think about how different your worst shift could feel if someone you respect took the time to help you unpack what happened, identify what you learned, and recognize how you grew stronger through the experience. That's the difference between feeling defeated and feeling prepared for whatever comes next.

The Knowledge Bridge

The right professional connection serves as a bridge between where you are and where you could be. They possess experience, skills, or insights that can accelerate your learning curve in ways that formal education alone cannot provide. These individuals don't just share technical expertise; they offer wisdom about navigating the complexities of healthcare culture, making strategic career decisions, and developing the confidence to advocate for yourself and your patients. They help you avoid common pitfalls while encouraging you to take calculated risks that move your career forward.

The Door Opener

This strategic connection possesses something invaluable: access to opportunities and networks that might otherwise remain invisible to you. They understand the unspoken pathways to advancement and aren't afraid to advocate for your potential.

These individuals make introductions that matter, recommend you for positions you might not have known existed, and help you gain visibility in ways that feel authentic rather than self-promotional. Their professional currency becomes partially yours, opening pathways that seemed permanently closed.

The power of this type of connection extends beyond immediate opportunities. When someone with credibility vouches for your potential, it changes how others perceive you and, more importantly, how you perceive yourself. You begin to see yourself as someone worthy of bigger challenges and greater responsibilities.

The Loving Challenger

The most transformative connections aren't always the most comfortable ones. The right person will challenge you to grow beyond your current limitations, even when that growth feels uncomfortable.

They see potential you're not ready to claim and push you toward opportunities that feel slightly beyond your reach. They encourage you to speak up in meetings, apply for positions that intimidate you, and take on responsibilities that stretch your capabilities.

Their belief in your potential often exceeds your own belief in yourself, and their gentle pressure helps you discover reserves of courage and competence you didn't know existed.

Research on growth mindset shows that individuals who embrace challenges and view failures as learning opportunities demonstrate greater resilience and achievement over time (Dweck, 2006[23], Mindset: The New Psychology of Success). The right connection helps you develop this mindset by reframing setbacks as stepping stones and encouraging you to see obstacles as opportunities for growth.

The Living Example

The most powerful connections embody the qualities and achievements you aspire to develop. They serve as tangible proof that your goals are achievable, your challenges are surmountable, and your dreams are worth pursuing. Watching someone navigate their career with integrity, resilience, and purpose provides a roadmap for your own journey. Their example answers the question that often keeps us stuck: "Is it really possible to have a fulfilling nursing career?"

Cultivating Your Freedom Network

Building meaningful professional relationships requires intentionality, but it doesn't require perfection. You don't need to be the most polished or confident person in the room. You simply need to be genuine, curious, and willing to step slightly outside your comfort zone.

The freedom you're seeking in nursing isn't about escaping to a different unit, getting that management position, or even leaving bedside altogether. The freedom you want—the ability to influence decisions, create opportunities, and practice nursing on your own terms—has been quietly waiting in the most overlooked aspect of our

---

[23] Dweck, C. (2006). Mindset: *The new psychology of success*. Random House.

profession: intentionally building a network of healthcare professionals who can collectively create the freedom you're seeking.

Waiting for that one right person to appear isn't a strategy. While that transformative connection matters deeply, professional relationships are so crucial to your freedom in nursing that building bridges to a collective community of people who can support, guide, and elevate your career is what actually changes your trajectory.

Most of us think of professional relationships as something formal, something that requires business cards and awkward small talk at conferences. Relationships that actually create freedom are far more organic, far more accessible, and probably already beginning to form around you. They can be found in the colleagues who share your frustrations, the nurses on social media who validate your experiences, the professionals in other departments who respect your expertise.

When we start building intentional professional relationships, we're not just networking—we're creating a collective map of the maze, finding shortcuts others have discovered, and building bridges over walls that seemed insurmountable when we faced them alone.

50 Ways to Build Your Freedom Network

1. **Start exactly where you are.** That nurse you always run into in the medication room? Strike up a real conversation beyond "crazy day, huh?" Ask about their path into bedside nursing. You might discover they share your sentiment of feeling trapped, and suddenly you have an ally and a solid book recommendation to share.

2. **Comment meaningfully on LinkedIn posts.** Not just "Great post!" but share your own experience with what they're discussing. This is how digital strangers become professional allies.

3. **Create a "Wins Wednesday" tradition on your unit** where everyone shares something that went well. Watch how celebrating together builds bonds that extend beyond work.

4. **Join that Facebook group for your specialty.** That's where thousands of nurses are solving the exact problems keeping you up at night.

5. **Become the unofficial unit photographer.** Document the good moments, the team victories, the holiday potlucks. Being the person who captures memories makes you memorable.

6. **Start a podcast—seriously.** Interview one nurse a month about their journey. You'll be shocked at how willing people are to share, and how those conversations transform into lasting connections.

7. **Volunteer to precept, but do it differently.** Take your orientee to lunch. Share your mistakes, not just your successes. These vulnerable moments create relationships that last entire careers.

8. **Write about your worst shift** (without patient identifiers, of course) and share it in a nursing forum. Shared struggles create instant bonds.

9. **Attend one conference a year.** Skip one session and hang out in the hallway. That's where real conversations happen, where business cards turn into coffee dates.

10. **Create a unit book club, but make it fun.** Read books about resilience, not just nursing theory. Meet at someone's house with wine. Professional development doesn't have to feel like homework.

11. **Teach something you're good at.** Maybe it's IV insertion, maybe it's dealing with difficult families. Becoming known for expertise in something specific draws people to you.

12. **Find nurses on TikTok or Instagram who make you laugh or think.** Consistently message them. Tell them their content matters. These digital relationships often become surprisingly real.

13. **Join your hospital committee that everyone complains about but no one joins.** Being one of the few who shows up gets you noticed by leadership—and not in a bad way.

14. **Become a mentor and flip the script.** Ask your mentee to teach you something too. The best professional relationships flow both ways.

15. **Start "Coffee with Random Colleague Fridays."** Once a month, have coffee with someone from a different department. The respiratory therapist, the social worker, the unit secretary. Expand your definition of professional network.

16. **Share your continuing education notes.** That expensive conference you attended? Send key takeaways to colleagues who couldn't go. Generosity builds loyalty.

17. **Create a WhatsApp group for night shift nurses at your hospital.** Being the connector who brings isolated people together makes you indispensable.

18. **Write LinkedIn articles about what you wish you'd known as a new nurse.** Your vulnerability will attract others who need to hear they're not alone.

19. **Volunteer for the holiday party planning.** It's how you meet nurses from every unit in a relaxed setting.

20. **Shadow a nurse in a completely different specialty for a day.** The NICU if you're ER. The OR if you're med-surg. These experiences create cross-unit relationships and might reveal hidden passions.

21. **Start a "Nurses Who Lift" group or walking club.** Combining fitness with professional connections creates bonds that extend beyond work topics.

22. **Become active in your specialty organization.** Volunteer to check people in at events. It forces you to meet everyone, and everyone remembers the friendly face at registration.

23. **Create a shared Google Doc of resources for your unit—** policies, tips, contact numbers. Being the resource creator makes you the go-to person.

24. **Reach out to that nurse author whose book you loved.** Tell them specifically what helped you. Authors remember readers who take time to connect.

25. **Start a monthly potluck for your shift.** Food brings people together like nothing else. The ICU nurse sharing their grandmother's recipe creates connection beyond work roles.

26. **Document and share your unit's innovations.** That new way you organized supplies? That communication system you developed? Write it up, share it widely. Innovation attracts innovators.

27. **Find your hospital's Facebook group** (the unofficial one where people really talk). Engage thoughtfully. Be helpful. Become known as someone who adds value, not drama.

28. **Attend grand rounds, even when the topic isn't directly relevant.** Ask one thoughtful question. Physicians remember nurses who engage intellectually.

29. **Create welcome packages for new hires on your unit.** Include personal notes from team members. Being the welcomer creates instant positive associations.

30. **Join Twitter or Threads nursing chats** (#NurseTwitter is real and active). The conversations happening there will blow your mind and expand your network globally.

31. **Organize "Lunch and Learn" sessions** where different nurses teach mini-lessons. The diabetic educator, the wound care specialist—everyone has expertise to share.

32. **Find three nurses whose careers you admire and ask them for 15-minute phone calls.** Most people are flattered and willing. These conversations can redirect your entire path.

33. **Create a "Difficult Case Debrief" group** that meets monthly to process challenging situations. The vulnerability required builds deep professional bonds.

34. **Volunteer for medical missions, local or international.** The intensity of these experiences creates lifelong professional relationships.

35. **Start writing thank-you notes to colleagues who helped during tough shifts.** Handwritten appreciation is so rare these days, it's memorable.

36. **Build relationships with nursing students during their rotations.** Today's student is tomorrow's colleague, and they remember who was kind.

37. **Connect with nurses in your community outside the hospital.** School nurses, clinic nurses, home health nurses. Your neighborhood is full of colleagues you haven't met.

38. **Become the unit champion for something**—falls prevention, pressure injuries, whatever interests you. Expertise attracts relationships.

39. **Create a "New Nurse Survival Guide" based on your experience.** Share it freely. Generosity with knowledge builds professional karma.

40. **Attend your hospital's research presentations.** Connect with nurse researchers. Your bedside observations might be their next study.

41. **Join online courses related to nursing interests.** The discussion boards become professional networking spaces.

42. **Start a "Skills Exchange" where nurses teach each other.** The ED nurse teaches emergency assessment skills, the ICU nurse teaches drips. Everyone wins.

43. **Document your journey on social media.** Your growth story attracts others on similar paths.

44. **Connect with nurses who've left bedside for alternative careers.** Their perspectives and connections open doors you didn't know existed.

45. **Participate in policy discussions at your hospital.** Being someone who thoughtfully engages with system issues gets you noticed by decision-makers.

46. **Create study groups for certifications.** The bonds formed while struggling through difficult material together last long after the test.

47. **Reach out to speakers after presentations with specific questions or comments.** Speakers remember engaged audience members.

48. **Build relationships with your nurse manager's network.** The managers who know your manager become aware of you by association.

49. **Share job opportunities you see, even if they're not for you.** Being the person who helps others advance builds incredible goodwill.

50. **Remember this: every nurse you meet is fighting their own battle with the maze.** When you approach relationships with empathy and authenticity, professional connections become personal freedoms.

The Truth About Professional Freedom

Professional relationships aren't really about networking at all. They're about finding your tribe within nursing. They're about discovering that you're not alone in feeling trapped, and more importantly, you're not alone in wanting more.

Every relationship you build is another rope thrown down into the maze, another ladder propped against the walls, another tunnel dug under the barriers. Some connections will become lifelong friendships. Others will be brief encounters that change your trajectory. You won't know which is which at first, and that's okay.

The freedom you're seeking—the autonomy, the sense of purpose— won't come from a single relationship or a perfect networking strategy. It will emerge from the web of connections you build, maintain, and nurture over time. Some days you'll be the one offering support. Other days you'll be the one needing it. That's how professional relationships create freedom: through the reciprocal flow of support, opportunity, and possibility.

Start where you are. Start with one conversation, one connection, one authentic interaction. The maze that feels so isolating right now? It's actually full of other nurses looking for the same freedom you are. When you start building bridges between each other, the walls don't seem quite so high anymore.

Somewhere in the maze, your future network holds the keys to the freedom you've been searching for—and perhaps the unique purpose you didn't know you were moving toward.

REFLECTION ACTIVITY:

Growing Your Professional Network

Before moving on, think about these questions:

- Who in your professional life has inspired or challenged you?

- Is there someone you've admired but haven't reached out to yet? What's stopping you?

- What steps can you take this week to build or strengthen a professional connection?

- If you could only implement five networking ideas from this chapter over the next 6 months, which five would create the most freedom in your career?

CHAPTER TEN

ONE STEP OUTSIDE

Breaking Free from Bedside Limitations

Every tree, every breeze whispers what our hospital routines often make us forget: you are free to step out.

Think back to a time when you've just finished your shift. The beeping monitors, hurried conversations, and perpetual chill of air conditioning and recycled air are behind you. The automatic doors slide open, and for a moment, you stand still. The evening air hits your face, cool and fresh, carrying a hint of something you hadn't noticed all day—life outside the walls.

This chapter is about that door—the one that leads out, not just from your shift, but from the mental maze of feeling stuck. When you step outside and let nature's arms wrap around you, something begins to shift. The world feels bigger, and so do your possibilities.

Nature has an unmatched way of widening our perspective. Trees that have weathered decades of storms remind you that resilience doesn't happen overnight. Rivers don't force their way forward—they flow around obstacles, carving new paths over time. Participants who took a 90-minute walk in nature showed decreased activity in the brain's subgenual prefrontal cortex, an area associated with rumination and negative thought patterns (Bratman et al., 2015)[24]. This neurological shift explains why stepping outside often feels like emerging from a fog of overwhelming thoughts.

Imagine standing under the open sky after hours spent under hospital lights. The vastness above you invites you to look beyond the immediate demands of your day. You begin to ask yourself questions you haven't had time to ask: What do I want beyond this moment? What's possible for me if I change how I see things?

Nature quiets the noise and invites reflection. Instead of solving problems in rapid succession, you let your mind drift to something bigger: your future.

The Calming Place

After a grueling shift, your nervous system is still on high alert—heart and mind racing, muscles tense. Even after clocking out, the weight of the day can linger. Nature serves as a biological reset button.

---

[24] Bratman, G. N., Hamilton, J. P., Hahn, K. S., Daily, G. C., & Gross, J. J. (2015). Nature experience reduces rumination and subgenual prefrontal cortex activation. *Proceedings of the National Academy of Sciences, 112*(28), 8567-8572. https://doi.org/10.1073/pnas.1510459112

Exposure to green space for as little as 20 minutes has been demonstrated to significantly reduce cortisol levels, the primary stress hormone associated with anxiety and burnout (Hunter et al., 2019)[25]. Participants who spent time in natural environments showed measurable improvements in heart rate variability, indicating enhanced parasympathetic nervous system activation—the body's natural relaxation response.

Nature thrives in balance: day and night, rain and sun, growth and rest. As nurses, we are often caught in a cycle of giving without pausing to receive. Nature teaches an important lesson: balance isn't a luxury; it's essential for survival.

Taking time to step outside isn't selfish; it's self-preservation. Whether it's a walk during your break, a quiet morning hike, or a moment to sit in your backyard, these moments replenish what the bedside takes. Nature invites creativity. Maybe it's the way sunlight filters through the branches or the rhythm of your footsteps on a trail. Immersion in natural settings for four days without technological access has been shown to produce a 50% improvement in creative problem-solving performance (Atchley et al., 2012)[26]. Natural environments promote a mental state called "soft fascination"—a

---

[25] Hunter, M. R., Gillespie, B. W., & Chen, S. Y. P. (2019). Urban nature experiences reduce stress in the context of daily life based on salivary biomarkers. *Frontiers in Psychology, 10,* 722. https://doi.org/10.3389/fpsyg.2019.00722

[26] Atchley, R. A., Strayer, D. L., & Atchley, P. (2012). Creativity in the wild: Improving creative reasoning through immersion in natural settings. *PLoS ONE, 7*(12), e51474. https://doi.org/10.1371/journal.pone.0051474

gentle engagement that allows the brain's default mode network to activate, facilitating innovative thinking and insight.

Have you ever noticed how the best ideas don't come when you're overthinking? They come when your mind wanders—on a walk, staring at the horizon, or listening to birds chirp at a park. In these quiet moments, your brain makes connections you didn't even know you were looking for. If you've felt stuck in the same routine, unsure how to move forward, remember: nature isn't static—it's alive, adaptive, and always growing. So are you. When you give yourself space to breathe and reflect, you open yourself to fresh ideas, new approaches, and unexpected solutions.

The Door Is Right in Front of You

You don't have to travel far to experience the healing power of nature. The path to clarity, peace, and renewed purpose begins the moment you choose to pause and step outside. Even hospital courtyards, small parks near your workplace, or simply sitting under a tree during your break can provide these benefits. The key isn't the perfect outdoor setting; it's your willingness to be present and allow nature to work its quiet magic on your overwhelmed system. That small garden area behind the medical center where you've rushed past countless times? What if you went there to have your lunch? It's waiting for you.

You don't need hiking boots, a weekend getaway, or even extra time in your schedule. You simply need to shift your awareness from rushing through these spaces to actually experiencing them. Instead of power walking to your car while mentally reviewing your shift, try walking slowly and noticing the sky above you. For those days when stepping outside isn't possible, even a view of nature through a window can provide benefits.

Studies have shown that patients with views of trees from their hospital rooms recover faster than those facing brick walls. The same principle applies to you. Taking a moment to gaze out at greenery, even through glass, can offer a mental reset that helps you approach the rest of your shift with renewed energy.

Make this practice intentional rather than accidental. Choose one outdoor space near your workplace that you'll visit regularly. Make it your consistent practice, just like washing your hands. This small commitment to yourself can become an anchor that keeps you grounded during the most demanding days.

Nature as Your Mirror: From Restoration to Rediscovery

Remember those trees that have weathered decades of storms, and those rivers that flow around obstacles rather than forcing their way forward? They teach us something vital about professional purpose. Just as nature demonstrates that resilience and adaptation aren't weaknesses but essential survival skills, your own career unfolds with the same wisdom. When you step outside after a shift and allow your mind to settle, you're not escaping your nursing practice—you're stepping into the same stance that nature takes: observing, adjusting, and flowing around what is slowing you down.

The clarity that emerges from these moments of reflection reveals something crucial: your unique purpose isn't found in pushing harder. Like the river carving new paths over time, your professional identity deepens and evolves through intentional pauses and the wisdom to recognize when you need to redirect your energy. When you return to the bedside with this restored perspective, you bring not just a calmer nervous system, but a renewed ability to recognize your unique purpose—to see where your practice aligns with your values and where you might need to carve a new path forward in your maze.

REFLECTION ACTIVITY:
Your Nature Escape Plan

Take a quiet moment to think about these questions:

- When was the last time you spent time in nature? How did it make you feel?

- What's one outdoor space nearby where you can go to reset after a shift?

- How can you build small nature breaks into your weekly or daily routine?

- What's one thing you'll focus on during your next walk—your breath, the sounds around you, or simply noticing your surroundings?

CHAPTER ELEVEN

THE MASTER KEY FOR BEDSIDE NURSES

Turning Your Know-How into Impact

Knowledge without action keeps you stuck; know-how applied creates freedom.

Nurses who successfully navigate their way out of feeling trapped at the bedside share one thing in common: they become obsessed with solving the right problem. These were specific problems that sat at the intersection of their unique expertise and their organization's genuine needs.

This chapter isn't about adding more tasks to your impossible schedule or learning another system that promises to fix everything. It's about recognizing that you already possess incredible know-how from your time in the maze—knowledge that could create measurable impact if you knew how to leverage it strategically.

Your Kobe Moment: Strategic Obsession

No one wants to compete against someone who is obsessed. Think Kobe. Kobe Bryant didn't simply play basketball with talent and effort; he approached the game with obsessive attention to detail. He studied game film with the intensity of a scholar, practiced shots that other players considered impossible until they became automatic, and approached every aspect of basketball with strategic focus that separated him from other incredibly talented athletes. His obsession wasn't random or scattered—it was strategically directed toward becoming unquestionably the best at the elements of the game that mattered most.

This is what happens when frontline expertise meets evidence-based thinking - and when a nurse refuses to just complain about a problem. When you align your unique know-how with strategic focus and a commitment to solving problems that create measurable impact, you stop competing on everyone else's terms and start playing a game that's tilted decisively in your favor.

Your bedside expertise means nothing if it's not strategically directed toward solving problems that matter to the people who have the power to create meaningful change within your organization. As we established in chapter seven, not every problem deserves your obsession. Strategic obsession means identifying problems that align with your unique know-how and have genuine potential to create measurable improvements in patient outcomes, staff satisfaction, or operational efficiency that your colleagues can recognize and value.

The Measurement Mindset

Not all problems within the bedside maze deserve your precious time. Many problems are highly visible and generate lots of discussion but have minimal impact on what actually matters for improving patient care or nurse retention. Others might operate under the radar but represent significant opportunities for improvement that could transform how your unit functions.

Your strategic obsession probably isn't hiding—it's the thing that's been staring you in the face every shift. It's the situation that has you explaining the same thing to patients over and over while thinking, "There has to be a better way to do this." It's the inefficiency that wastes your time every single shift while you mentally redesign the entire system.

You've found a problem worth obsessing over when solutions keep interrupting your thoughts. While your colleagues vent about the problem and move on, you find yourself sketching out ideas on napkins during your break. The problem meant for you to solve is the one where you naturally think, "I could fix this if someone would just let me try."

Developing what I call the measurement mindset transitions you from the person with good suggestions to the person who drives change that gets measured, funded, and promoted. *The measurement mindset starts with asking different questions.*

Instead of:

> ➤ Why can't they just fix this?
> ➤ This place is falling apart

> ➤ Nobody listens to us

> ➤ We're always short-staffed

You start asking:

> ➤ How would I measure if this process actually improved?

> ➤ What would success look like in numbers that matter to my hospital?

> ➤ Which metrics would change if we solved this problem?

> ➤ How could I prove this solution works?

Every healthcare organization obsesses over certain metrics because they directly impact patient outcomes, regulatory compliance, or financial performance. Your strategic obsession needs to connect to one of these metrics if you want to create change that gets noticed and supported.

Consider the data that keeps hospital leaders awake at night:

> ➤ Approximately 20% of Medicare beneficiaries are readmitted within 30 days, with research showing that 27% of these readmissions are potentially preventable ("Hospital Readmissions," StatPearls Publishing, January 2024)[27]. *If your obsession involves patient education or discharge planning, you're targeting a problem with massive financial and clinical implications.*

---

[27] StatPearls Publishing. (2024, June 7). Reducing Hospital Readmissions. In StatPearls [Internet]. Treasure Island (FL): StatPearls Publishing. Retrieved from https://www.ncbi.nlm.nih.gov/books/NBK606114/

➤ Medication errors occur in 6.5 per 100 hospital admissions ("Medication Errors," StatPearls Publishing, January 2024)[28][29]. *If your obsession centers on medication safety, systematic thinking, or catching details others miss, you're focusing on a problem that directly impacts patient safety and organizational liability.*

➤ Healthcare-associated infections affect approximately 1 in 31 hospital patients on any given day, with recent CDC data showing ongoing challenges despite prevention efforts ("HAI Prevalence Survey," CDC National and State Healthcare-Associated Infections Progress Report, 2024)[30]. **If your obsession involves infection prevention, environmental controls, or patient care protocols, you're targeting a problem with life-and-death implications.**

➤ The average cost of nurse turnover increased to $61,110 per departing RN in 2024, up from $56,300 in 2023, with each percent change in RN turnover costing or saving the average hospital $289,000 per year (NSI Nursing Solutions, Inc., "2024 National Health Care Retention & RN Staffing Report")[31]. **If your obsession involves workflow efficiency, nurse satisfaction, or**

---

[28] StatPearls Publishing. (2024, February 12). Medical Error Reduction and Prevention. In StatPearls [Internet]. Treasure Island (FL): StatPearls Publishing. Retrieved from https://www.ncbi.nlm.nih.gov/books/NBK499956/

[29] StatPearls Publishing. (2024, February 12). Medication Dispensing Errors and Prevention. In StatPearls [Internet]. Treasure Island (FL): StatPearls Publishing. Retrieved from https://www.ncbi.nlm.nih.gov/books/NBK519065/

[30] Centers for Disease Control and Prevention. (2024). Current HAI Progress Report. Retrieved from https://www.cdc.gov/healthcare-associated-infections/php/data/progress-report.html

[31] NSI Nursing Solutions. (2024). 2024 NSI National Health Care Retention & RN Staffing Report. Retrieved from https://www.nsinursingsolutions.com/Documents/Library/NSI_National_Health_Care_Retention_Report.pdf

creating better working conditions, you're addressing a problem that directly impacts your organization's bottom line and ability to provide quality care.

The measurement mindset means thinking about your obsession in terms of concrete, trackable outcomes. How would you measure success? What baseline data would you need to collect? How would you demonstrate that your solution actually works? What metrics would convince skeptical leaders that your idea deserves investment and support?

How One ICU Nurse Transformed Patient Safety

Every shift, she noticed the same problem: patients at highest risk weren't getting the consistent care they needed. As an intensive care nurse, she understood that her most vulnerable patients—those on critical medications and life support—faced a silent threat that nobody was systematically addressing. Hospital-acquired pressure injuries weren't just uncomfortable; they represented preventable harm in a population that already faced overwhelming odds.

Instead of complaining about the gap, she did something different. She dove into the research, reading peer-reviewed literature and studying what other facilities had tried. What she discovered was elegant in its simplicity: a structured turning protocol could work, but only if the burden was distributed fairly across the nursing team. The solution required systematic thinking, not heroic individual effort.

She proposed what became known as the "Turning Team"—a rotating assignment system where each nurse would take responsibility for repositioning all high-risk patients during their designated time slot. No more hoping someone would remember. No more competing priorities crushing essential care. Just clear accountability and shared responsibility.

The rollout was straightforward but deliberate. Training happened across all units. Visual management tools appeared on whiteboards. A dedicated support person was hired. Nurses got flexible scheduling options so they could choose slots that worked for their shifts.

The system accounted for real life—if someone got slammed with an emergency, colleagues could swap shifts or the charge nurse could step in.

Within weeks, something unexpected happened. Collaboration improved. Nurses appreciated knowing their high-risk patients would be turned consistently. The burden that once fell on individual nurses got distributed across the team. Metrics improved dramatically, with measurable reductions in pressure injuries appearing in the data.

What started as one nurse's obsession about a problem became a unit-wide transformation, then spread to the entire organization. Her colleagues didn't resist—they embraced it because the solution actually made their work better, not just more complicated.

This is what happens when frontline expertise meets evidence-based thinking. This is a real example of a nurse who successfully developed and implemented this turning team initiative at a major academic health system.

Taking Action: Powerful Questions for Your Strategic Obsession

Understanding these principles intellectually is one thing; applying them to your specific situation requires honest self-reflection. Take some time to consider these questions. Don't rush your answers. The goal isn't to have everything figured out immediately, but to begin the process of intentional career development.

> ➤ **What aspect of your current job energizes you rather than drains you?** Think beyond the obvious answers—maybe it's not direct patient care that lights you up, but the moment when you help a confused family member finally understand their loved one's treatment plan.

> ➤ **When do you feel most competent and confident in your abilities?** These moments reveal where your natural talents intersect with nursing skills.

> ➤ **What type of problems do you naturally gravitate toward solving on your floor?** Do you find yourself drawn to workflow inefficiencies, communication breakdowns, patient education gaps, or something else entirely? The problems that consistently catch your attention are signals pointing toward your natural area of interest.

> ➤ **What steps could you take to become an expert in your chosen area of focus?** Think beyond formal education— though that might be part of it. Consider shadowing experts,

volunteering for related committees, conducting informal research projects, or seeking out challenging cases that would stretch your abilities.

➤ **Who could you learn from that has developed expertise in this area?** These might be people within your organization or experts you discover through professional organizations, conferences, or literature. Don't overlook the possibility of reaching out to people whose work you admire—many experts are more accessible than you might think.

➤ **What resources could help you go deeper?** Books, courses, conferences, and mentorship opportunities are obvious choices, but also consider podcasts, online communities, research journals, professional associations, and certification programs. The key is developing a systematic approach to building your solutions rather than random learning.

➤ **What problems in your workplace align with your unique know-how?** Identify where your unique know-how as discussed in chapter six intersects with your organization's genuine needs. This is your sweet spot—where your distinctive combination of skills, passion, and perspective can create measurable impact.

➤ **How could you measure the impact of solving these problems?** Think like a hospital administrator or quality improvement specialist. What metrics would demonstrate that your solution works? How would you collect baseline data and track progress over time?

> ➤ **Who are the decision-makers who would care about these improvements?** Identifying the right stakeholders is crucial for gaining support and resources. These might be nurse managers, quality directors, chief nursing officers, or even physicians who influence how things work on your unit.

How to Turn Your Know-How Into Opportunity

Before you approach your manager, identify one specific problem or gap on your unit that aligns with your unique know-how.

Don't just say "I want to go to a conference" or "I want to lead something."

Consider framing your observation as "I've noticed [**specific problem**], and based on my strengths in [**your skill**], passion for [**what energizes you**], and perspective on [**how you see things differently**], I believe I could [**solve this problem/improve this process/lead this initiative**]."

Here's a way to frame your proposal:

> ➤ **What you're asking for:** "I'd like to [attend X conference/lead Y project/pilot Z initiative]"

> ➤ **What the unit gets:** "This would directly address [the problem you identified] and result in [specific outcome]"

> ➤ **What you'll deliver:** "Within [timeframe], I'll [concrete deliverable—training for staff, new protocol, presentation of what you learned]"

Example: *"I've noticed our new grads struggle with time management during their first few months, which impacts the whole team. Given my strengths in workflow planning and my passion for teaching, I'd like to pilot a 30-day mentorship structure where I guide two new grads through organizing their shifts. At the end of 30 days, I'll present what worked to the leadership team so we can use it and show other unit leaders if it's effective."*

When you combine obsession triggers, measurement mindset, and a focus on solutions, you develop a strategic advantage in the maze. Problems that once felt like intimidating roadblocks become new pathways packed with purpose.

When you're working toward solving a problem you genuinely care about, work that once felt meaningless starts feeling more meaningful.

Strategic obsession transforms you from someone trapped by problems into someone who creates solutions.

By becoming the person who solves what everyone else just complains about, you don't just find your way out—you can discover your unique purpose within bedside nursing. This is how you move from feeling trapped at the bedside to finding unexpected meaning in the work only you can do.

This is your Kobe moment within the bedside maze. Take advantage of it.

Additional Supporting Sources:

➢ Agency for Healthcare Research and Quality. (2024, April 19). Clinical Conditions With Frequent, Costly Hospital Readmissions by Payer, 2020. HCUP Statistical Brief #307. Retrieved from https://hcup-us.ahrq.gov/reports/statbriefs/sb307-readmissions-2020.jsp

➢ Becker's Hospital Review. (2024, April 7). The cost of nurse turnover in 24 numbers. Retrieved from https://www.beckershospitalreview.com/finance/the-cost-of-nurse-turnover-in-24-numbers-2024/

➢ South Florida Hospital News. (2024). Creation of the patient turning team: A clinical nurse-led initiative for pressure injury prevention. Retrieved from https://southfloridahospitalnews.com/creation-of-the-patient-turning-team-a-clinical-nurse-led-initiative-for-pressure-injury-prevention/

YOUR UNIQUE CLARITY

CHAPTER TWELVE

THE CEO MINDSET

Becoming the CEO of Your Nursing Career

You're not just an employee—you're the chief executive of your future.

Sarah had been a bedside nurse for eight years when she found herself sitting across from a healthcare start-up executive recruiter. The recruiter outlined a leadership role partnering with a prestigious health system and described what they needed: someone who could manage complex operations, coordinate multiple stakeholders, handle crisis situations, and drive quality outcomes under pressure.

Sarah felt her heart sink. "I don't have that kind of experience," she said. "I'm *just* a bedside nurse."

The recruiter looked at her strangely. "Sarah, you've been managing a $3 million annual patient load, coordinating care across multiple departments, responding to emergencies weekly, and maintaining satisfaction scores in the 95th percentile. You were highly recommended by your nursing leaders."

Sarah's response reveals something critical: She wasn't lacking in CEO-level capability. She was lacking in CEO-level thinking.

The difference between the average bedside nurse and a nurse who thinks like a CEO isn't competence—it's ownership.

A CEO understands their role within a larger organizational context. They make strategic decisions about priorities and resources. They communicate their value. They build visibility around their impact. They deliberately position themselves for their future. Most bedside nurses don't. They show up, do excellent work, and wait for someone to recognize it.

The CEO Mindset: 3 Pillars to Owning Your Nursing Career

Pillar 1: Strategic Value

A CEO never stops asking: "What value am I creating and how does it translate to organizational outcomes?"

Most bedside nurses don't frame their work this way. You think: "I took care of my patients." A CEO would think: "I prevented two complications that would have cost thousands in additional care, coordinated care across three departments in a way that shortened the patient's length of stay by a day, and maintained satisfaction scores that protect the hospital's reputation."

Both statements describe the same work. One is invisible. One is strategic.

Sarah managed a $3 million patient load. That's not a random number. That's the total annual cost of caring for her patients—ICU stays, surgical costs, pharmacy, diagnostics, and all the associated expenses. When you prevent a complication that would have extended a patient's stay by three days, you're directly impacting that number. You're not just "doing your job." You're creating measurable value.

Strategic value means understanding what matters to your organization and how your work contributes to it.

Your organization cares about:

- Patient outcomes (mortality, complications, readmissions)
- Patient satisfaction (HCAHPS scores, Net Promoter Score)
- Staff retention (turnover costs money)
- Operational efficiency (length of stay, throughput, resource utilization)
- Regulatory compliance (avoiding citations, maintaining accreditation)
- Financial performance (revenue, costs, margin)

Everything you do at the bedside touches one or more of these. The CEO mindset is this: "I create value across multiple organizational departments. I should think clearly about what that value is, measure it when possible, and communicate it when necessary."

Pillar 2: Visibility

A CEO makes sure their impact is seen. This isn't about self-promotion or boasting. It's about accurate visibility. If you do something that no one knows about, it has zero impact on your career trajectory. That's not fair—but it's true.

Think about how visibility works at the executive level. CEOs give quarterly earnings calls. They publish annual reports. They speak at conferences. They make sure key stakeholders know what's being accomplished. They do this not because they're arrogant, but because visibility is how impact becomes credible. Bedside nurses almost never do this. You do extraordinary work and document it in ways that make it sound ordinary. Your shift notes read like every other competent nurse's shift notes. That documentation is invisible. It's fine for clinical purposes, but it's terrible for visibility of your actual impact.

Consider these visibility strategies that extend beyond typical hospital committee work:

> **Creating intellectual property from your know-how:** What if your expertise didn't just live in your head? Imagine writing a one-page protocol for managing a specific patient population. What if that framework became something other nurses used?

> **Building visibility outside your organization:** What if your expertise wasn't limited to your hospital walls? Consider what happens when you share your work more broadly. You might write an article for a nursing journal about what you learned. You could present at a regional nursing conference about your approach to a specific challenge. Some nurses create podcast content or video demonstrations. What if nurses across the country knew your work?

> ➤ **Creating new bedside processes:** What if you didn't just do the existing job better, but expanded what the job could be? Consider where the system has gaps. Created a new workflow? Invented a new approach to patient care or consistent family communication? Imagine proposing something that doesn't currently exist and it later becomes the gold standard for direct patient care.

A CEO doesn't chase attention. They create it with intention.

Pillar 3: Intentional Positioning

A CEO makes strategic choices about where they position themselves in the organization.

Most bedside nurses don't think strategically about positioning. You take the job you're offered and do it well. You respond to opportunities when they come. You don't actively shape where you are and where you're headed. A CEO thinks differently: "What positions would allow me to leverage my expertise"?

Intentional positioning means making choices about:

> ➤ **Where you work within bedside nursing.** Not all bedside nursing roles are the same. Some units are innovative and oriented toward professional development. Others are traditional and focused on volume. Some have strong nursing leadership. Others don't. A CEO would choose deliberately—not just taking the first job available, but thinking about where their expertise would be valued and where they could grow.

➢ **How you communicate about your future.** Do your leaders know what matters to you? Do you talk about where you want to go? Or do you just work hard and hope someone notices? A CEO has explicit conversations about trajectory. You tell your manager: "I'm interested in clinical leadership roles. Here's what I'm building toward. Here's how I want to develop." You don't wait for an opportunity to come to you. You make it visible.

➢ **What role you play in your organization.** Are you someone who complains about problems or solves them? Are you someone who resists change or leads it? Are you someone who maintains the status quo or improves it? A CEO positions themselves as a value creator, not a task executor. You show up as someone who thinks about the bigger picture, not just your individual patient assignment.

When you start thinking like a CEO, you stop waiting for recognition and start creating it. Begin exploring new ways to add strategic value, increase your visibility, and position yourself intentionally—because your influence at the bedside grows the moment you decide to lead your career instead of letting it lead you.

I've shared examples for each pillar, but the real power comes when you start seeing new possibilities on your own. Keep challenging yourself to find creative ways to apply the CEO mindset in each career decision you make.

Executive Leadership: Your CEO Toolkit

Sarah didn't need to develop new capabilities to qualify for that leadership role. She needed to recognize and articulate the executive-level capabilities she'd already been developing through bedside nursing. I don't want what happened to her to happen to you. You've been developing executive capabilities every single shift without even realizing it. Let me walk you through what you've actually been mastering—with the real bedside work that proves it.

Crisis Command: Emergency Response Leadership

You're three hours into your shift when your patient's oxygen saturation drops from 94% to 78% in four minutes. No clear reason. You're immediately assessing—is it the new medication? Equipment failure? Aspiration? You call the physician, alert respiratory, position the patient, gather the equipment, and coordinate the response while keeping the family from panicking and ensuring the other patients on your team don't get neglected.

Within minutes, you've made critical decisions, coordinated multiple departments, and prevented a code situation.

This is what executives study in crisis management courses. You do it before lunch.

Stakeholder Navigation: Managing Competing Demands

A family member wants their mother discharged today. The physician says she needs 48 more hours of care. The patient is confused about what she actually needs. The case manager is focused on bed availability. Insurance is questioning the length of stay.

You're the one translating between all of them—helping the family understand why discharge isn't safe yet without making them feel unheard, supporting the physician's clinical judgment, advocating for what the patient actually needs, and keeping the care plan moving forward. You hold all these competing perspectives without fracturing the team or abandoning anyone's legitimate concerns.

That's complex multi-stakeholder relationship management.

Clinical Synthesis: Diagnostic Pattern Recognition

Your patient's labs look fine. Vital signs are stable. But something feels off. You've seen this pattern before—the subtle restlessness, the way she's breathing, the color of her skin. You trust that pattern more than the numbers and call the physician back. It's a developing infection. Three hours later, antibiotics are working. You synthesized incomplete, sometimes contradictory information and made a clinical judgment that protocols alone wouldn't have caught.

That's complex data analysis and decision-making under uncertainty— the exact skill that distinguishes executive-level thinking.

Difficult Conversation Mastery: Crisis Communication

The family is angry. Their mother fell during the night shift and fractured her hip. You're delivering news they don't want to hear, in a moment when they're terrified and looking for someone to blame.

You maintain professionalism and compassion simultaneously. You explain what happened without making excuses.

You answer their questions honestly. You demonstrate institutional competence even in a failure. By the end of the conversation, they feel heard instead of adversarial. That conversation either becomes a litigation risk or a story they tell about how the hospital handled a difficult situation with integrity.

That's customer relations during crisis situations—the kind of emotional intelligence that separates organizations that generate complaints from ones that maintain reputation.

Resourcefulness: Making Excellence Happen With Less

You're short-staffed. The patient census is high. The acuity is higher than normal. You have fewer supplies than ideal and equipment is aging. Yet you still deliver quality care, prevent complications, and maintain patient satisfaction. You prioritize ruthlessly. You work efficiently. You make your resources stretch further than the organizational model suggests should be possible. You're the reason your department doesn't collapse when budgets get cut.

You're operating at the efficiency level executives are hired to create.

Informal Authority: Leadership Without a Title

The patient needs wound care, but the wound care nurse is on another unit. The physician needs labs drawn stat, but the lab tech is backed up. The family needs someone to explain the treatment plan, but the doctor is in surgery.

You're coordinating physicians, specialists, therapists, and support staff who don't report to you—people over whom you have zero formal authority. Yet the work gets coordinated. The care aligns. The patient's needs get met. You've prevented the coordination breakdowns that typically cause errors.

That's informal leadership across hierarchies—the skill that makes complex organizations actually work.

Patient Education: Behavior Change That Sticks

Your diabetic patient nods along when you explain blood sugar monitoring, but you recognize he's not actually understanding it. You switch approaches—you show him the exact process, have him demonstrate it back to you, explain why it matters in language that connects to his life. You teach in a way that actually sticks. He leaves understanding not just what to do, but why it matters and how to do it in his real life. His compliance improves. His readmissions decrease. His outcomes improve.

You're operating at the level of adult education and behavior change facilitation—the skill that transforms knowledge into action.

Financial Stewardship: Cost-Conscious Clinical Decision-Making

Every decision you make—the dressing you choose, whether to use a certain intervention, how you manage preventable complications— affects organizational revenue and costs. You understand this intuitively.

You prevent unnecessary procedures. You reduce complications that extend length of stay. You improve outcomes that directly impact reimbursement rates. You're not making decisions based on cost alone, but you're making decisions with cost awareness built in.

That's financial impact management at the clinical level.

How the CEO Mindset Elevates You in the Maze

Most nurses navigate the bedside maze reactively—hoping someone notices. A nurse with a CEO mindset navigates it differently. They don't try to escape. They own it.

Here's how I did it.

When I started Med-Surg RN PRO, I wasn't abandoning bedside nursing—I was expanding how I showed up as **a leader**. I was thinking strategically about the problems I saw every shift, solving them systematically. My colleagues didn't see me as just another competent nurse anymore. They saw someone building something, thinking bigger, and creating solutions. I became the person others wanted to follow—not because I had a title, but because I was thinking and acting outside the box.

Med-Surg RN PRO positioned me as valuable in ways that mattered. I became visible as someone with expertise, someone building innovative solutions, someone transforming how nurses experience their work. I wasn't interchangeable anymore. People recognized what I was building. That visibility created **opportunities** I couldn't have accessed by just being a good bedside nurse.

Every challenge at the bedside—the workflow inefficiencies, the nurse burnout, the impossible scheduling—stopped being problems that happened to me. They became the raw material for solutions I was building. The maze wasn't something I was trapped in. It was the foundation of everything I was creating. That shift in **perspective** changed alot about my relationship to work.

Instead of choosing between bedside nursing and something away from the bedside, I created a third pathway. I maintained my clinical practice while building Med-Surg RN PRO. I developed specialized expertise that made me valuable in multiple areas of nursing.

This one decision now gives me value at the bedside and away from the bedside. I could mentor nurses, speak to groups, develop digital and physical products, run a business—all while staying connected to the bedside that grounded everything I did. The maze didn't change, but my options multiplied **exponentially**.

I stopped waiting for someone to recognize my potential and started building. I identified the problems I was uniquely positioned to solve. I built relationships with people who understood what I was creating. I made intentional choices about where to invest my energy. I created my own pathway instead of following someone else's.

The maze hasn't changed, but you have. Your CEO mindset is stronger, your vision is clearer, and I am proof that you can become the CEO of your nursing career.

Visit **medsurgrnpro.com** to see what's possible when you stop asking permission and start building a new pathway in the maze using strategic value, visibility, intentional positioning, and your unique purpose.

REFLECTION ACTIVITY:
The CEO Mindset

- **Think about your most challenging shift in the past month.** List three specific situations where you made decisions, solved problems, or coordinated resources. For each situation, rewrite it using business language instead of nursing language.

- **If you had to present your nursing experience to a hospital board as qualifications for a leadership position, what would be your top three accomplishments?** Write each accomplishment in terms of measurable impact: What problems did you solve? What outcomes did you improve? What resources did you manage effectively?

CHAPTER THIRTEEN

THE PROFESSIONAL MIRROR

How Feedback Reflects Your Path to Excellence

A nurse who ignores feedback will stay stuck in the same hallway forever.

What if the most uncomfortable conversation you have this week is the key to becoming the nurse you've always wanted to be?

You're walking to your car after a brutal twelve-hour shift. You saved a life tonight—literally prevented someone from coding through your quick thinking and advocacy. You're exhausted but proud. Then your phone buzzes.

A text from your manager: "Can we talk tomorrow about your documentation? A few things to discuss." Your heart sinks. After everything you accomplished tonight, after pouring your soul into patient care, someone wants to critique your charting. The pride you felt moments ago transforms into defensiveness. Your mind races through justifications: "I was busy saving lives, not pushing papers."

Mirrors don't lie, even when the reflection is uncomfortable. The nurses who transition from good to extraordinary aren't the ones who avoid these reflections. They're the ones who lean into the discomfort and ask, "What if there's something here I need to see?"

If the bedside is a maze, then feedback is like having strategically placed mirrors throughout that maze. Some mirrors reflect your victories—showing you moments when your nursing excellence shines brightest. Others reflect your blind spots—revealing pathways to improvement you couldn't see from your current position. Some simply show you exactly where you are, helping you navigate toward where you want to be.

Most of us have learned to avoid these mirrors or, worse, to interpret every reflection as personal criticism. We've been conditioned to see feedback as judgment rather than guidance, as attack rather than assistance in finding our way through the professional maze.

Feedback isn't another obstacle in the bedside maze—it's the navigation system that helps you discover those unexpected paths to your unique nursing purpose.

The Three Types of Professional Mirrors

Think of every piece of feedback as one of three different mirrors, each showing you something unique about your journey through the nursing maze. In their book *Thanks for the Feedback*, Stone and Heen (2014)[32] explain that effective feedback falls into three categories—appreciation, coaching, and evaluation—each serving a different purpose in professional development. Understanding which mirror you're looking into helps you interpret what you're seeing more accurately.

The Appreciation Mirror: Seeing Your Impact When You Can't See It Yourself

You know those moments when a colleague thanks you for staying late to help, or when a family specifically asks for you to care for their loved one? That's the appreciation mirror reflecting your impact. This mirror shows you exactly when your nursing purpose shines brightest.

This isn't just about warm feelings. The appreciation mirror reveals the specific moments when you're fulfilling your deepest calling as a nurse. When someone told me that my calm presence during a crisis helped them feel safe, I realized they were showing me how my commitment to practicing emotional intelligence as a deliberate skill translates into actual patient safety. I remember early in my career—those moments during an RRT when I wanted to leave my patient's room and hide in the supply room. Back then, I wasn't calm. I wasn't reflective. I didn't understand how my own anxiety and body

---

[32] Stone, D., & Heen, S. (2014). Thanks for the feedback: The science and art of receiving feedback well. Viking.

language affected the people around me. But when patients and colleagues started acknowledging how my presence steadied them during chaotic moments, I realized something had shifted. I had become more self-aware about my reactions, more intentional about my composure, and more reflective about how I showed up during emergencies. That feedback was proof of my growth—from a nurse running from the intensity to a nurse who could sit in it with clarity.

When a new nurse sought my guidance, they reflected something equally important back to me. It became clear that connecting with the next generation of bedside nurses wasn't just something I naturally did—it was something I needed to do more of, not less. Every time a newer nurse asked for help, I viewed it as my responsibility to pass forward what I'd learned. Those moments became less about answering questions and more about building the kind of mentor relationship that prevents nurses from ever feeling like they need to hide.

Most nurses dismiss appreciation feedback as "just being nice." This mirror is showing you your professional superpowers in action. This feedback reveals the aspects of your nursing practice that create the most healing, the most impact, and the most trust.

The Coaching Mirror: Illuminating Your Growth Edge

Your nurse manager says, "I noticed you seemed overwhelmed during the staff meeting yesterday. Want to talk about some strategies for staying centered when things get intense?"

This is the coaching mirror, and yes, it can sting a little. Think of this feedback as reflecting not your flaws, but your growth edges—the places where your nursing practice is ready to expand. The person holding up this mirror isn't questioning your heart for nursing; they're showing you the gap between where you are and where your commitment to patient care is moving you toward.

In the bedside maze, coaching feedback is like someone pointing out a pathway you hadn't noticed before. The suggestion might feel uncomfortable because it requires you to change direction or try something new, but it's actually showing you routes to becoming more effective at what you care about most.

The coaching mirror reflects specific skills that, when you develop them, make you better at fulfilling your mission to serve patients during their most vulnerable moments. The reflection you see might be uncomfortable, but it's showing you exactly where your growth can have the biggest impact on the outcomes that matter to you.

I learned this the hard way as a charge nurse. I approached a nurse in the medication room to talk about something I'd observed—she consistently asked for help at the end of her shift, and I thought she needed to hear that directly. My delivery was straightforward. What I didn't realize was that my tone, my matter-of-factness, had landed like a gut punch. She stood there in the medication room, and tears started running down her face.

When she found words to explain what happened, she told me something I couldn't argue with: my words and my tone had made her feel exactly like her father had when she was a child. Small. Criticized. Unsafe.

That stung. It still stings to write it. But instead of defending my approach, I chose to see her feedback as a coaching mirror reflecting exactly where I needed to grow as a leader. This wasn't about softening my standards or accepting mediocrity. It was about recognizing that how I delivered feedback mattered as much as what I said. My straightforwardness without consideration for her emotional safety wasn't leadership—it was just harshness dressed up as honesty.

She never escalated this moment to management. Instead, she trusted me with her vulnerability, which meant I had to earn that trust by actually changing. That moment taught me to pause before speaking, to consider my tone as carefully as my words, and to lead with the understanding that people remember how you made them feel far longer than they remember what you said.

Today, every time I give feedback, I carry that moment with me. It made me a better leader.

The Evaluation Mirror: Reflecting Your Professional Standing

Annual reviews, competency assessments, performance evaluations—these formal feedback sessions can feel the most threatening because they often come with consequences. The evaluation mirror serves a crucial purpose in helping you stay on the pathways that lead to professional excellence. In the bedside maze, evaluation feedback is like checkpoint mirrors that confirm you're still on track toward your professional destination. Sometimes these mirrors show you that you need to adjust your route slightly to stay aligned with the standards that protect both your patients and your career.

Early in my career, a nurse manager told me she saw supervisor potential in me. If I committed to earning a certification or enrolled in a graduate nursing program, she'd strongly consider me for a nurse supervisor position that would open soon. It was validation of my performance—and it was also a fork in the road. I had to pause and ask myself a hard question: Did I want to go that route?

The answer was no. Not because I wasn't capable. Not because I didn't value professional advancement and leadership. I simply valued something else more—my four days off a week, traveling with my wife, the flexibility to pursue entrepreneurial projects, to serve on nonprofit boards, to contribute to my church, to leave work at work.

My evaluation mirror showed me I was a consistent high performer with leadership qualities at the bedside, and that was exactly where I wanted to be performing. Other nurses passed me on the traditional career ladder, and I stayed put. Intentionally.

I continued to meet every professional standard. I took on projects. I grew clinically. But I used each evaluation not as a directive to climb higher, but as a checkpoint showing me how close I was to the professional destination I had actually chosen for myself. The mirror wasn't telling me I was on the wrong path. It was confirming I was exactly where I needed to be at the moment.

Evaluation isn't about perfection—it's about progression. The reflection you see is a snapshot of where you are now, not a verdict on your worth as a nurse.

Don't Let the Messenger Distract from the Message

One of the biggest mistakes nurses make with feedback is getting so focused on how it's delivered—that they miss what it could teach them about better serving their patients. In professional relationships, some people are better at holding up mirrors than others.

This became clear to me one day at the bedside. I attempted to insert an NG tube on a patient and failed twice. I notified the well-known colorectal surgeon overseeing the patient. He was condescending about it. He interrupted what I was doing with other patients, came to the bedside with fresh supplies and a larger bore tube, and inserted it successfully while making it clear that my technique had been inadequate. His tone wasn't nice. His delivery was dismissive.

But when I looked past how he made me feel, I found something valuable: his approach—having the patient focus on the rhythm of swallow and breathe, swallow and breathe—created a smoother insertion than the method I'd been using. It wasn't that my technique was fundamentally wrong. It was that his refined approach worked better. I could have focused on his arrogance and missed it entirely. Instead, I extracted the practical skill and started using his method. That's what mattered.

The messenger was problematic, but the message had merit.

If there are established processes for accountability to address consistently poor communication, by all means use them. This is your challenge in navigating the maze: Can you separate the gold from the dirt? Can you find useful information even when it's wrapped in unprofessional delivery? Can you extract the navigation data you need to find your unique path even when the person providing the data lacks good mirror-holding skills? The goal isn't to become a doormat or to accept every piece of feedback as gospel truth. The goal is to maintain your ability to navigate professional relationships while staying focused on what serves you and your patients best.

Building Your Personal Feedback Navigation System

Create a personal process for handling feedback that keeps you connected to your nursing purpose while helping you navigate the professional maze more effectively:

- **Listen First:** Focus on understanding rather than defending. Ask questions that help you see how the feedback relates to patient care and outcomes. Treat the feedback conversation like a patient assessment—gather all the information before drawing conclusions.

- **Plan Action:** Develop specific steps for applying useful feedback, always connecting these steps to improved patient care. What one small change could you make that would address the feedback while enhancing your effectiveness?

- **Reflect Later:** Process the feedback away from the immediate situation. How does the feedback connect to your goals as a nurse and your commitment to excellence? What patterns do you notice in the feedback you receive? What pathways in the maze might this feedback be pointing toward?

➤ **Follow Up:** When appropriate, circle back to show how you've applied the input and demonstrate your commitment to growth. This builds trust and often results in more helpful feedback in the future.

Your Feedback Challenge

Here's your challenge: The next time you receive feedback—whether appreciation, coaching, or evaluation—pause before you react.

When someone appreciates your work, use that mirror to understand what you should do more of. When someone coaches you toward improvement, use that mirror to see pathways to greater effectiveness.

When someone evaluates your performance, use that mirror to assess your alignment with the standards that move you faster through your maze.

Your patients are counting on your willingness to grow. Your profession needs nurses who can receive feedback gracefully and use it to become more effective. You deserve to discover the pathways through the maze that lead to your unique purpose in nursing. The mirrors are already there, reflecting information that could transform your practice and accelerate your professional growth. Are you ready to look into them with curiosity instead of defensiveness? Are you ready to let feedback guide you toward becoming the nurse you've always wanted to be?

Your unique nursing purpose reveals itself not in avoiding feedback, but in how you transform that feedback into better care for those who need you most. The unexpected path to your nursing purpose might just begin with the feedback you've been avoiding.

CHAPTER FOURTEEN

SUCCESS REDEFINED

Considering Your Unique Career Path

Success is not a title—it's alignment with your purpose.

Every time you clock in for another shift, you're continuing a story that began over 160 years ago. This isn't just your career we're talking about—it's your opportunity for global impact. Understanding where nursing has been doesn't just give you perspective on where it's going. It reveals something profound about the unique role you're meant to play in this ongoing narrative.

Florence Nightingale didn't set out to revolutionize healthcare when she arrived in the Crimea in 1854. She simply saw an intolerable situation and refused to accept it as unchangeable. The mortality rate stood at a staggering 42%. Within six months, she had reduced that number to 2%. She didn't just save lives—she proved that nurses could be agents of systemic change.

Her greatest contribution wasn't the lamp or these statistics. It was the idea that nursing expertise could challenge traditional healthcare when nurses have a voice. She established the precedent that nurses don't just follow orders—they use clinical judgment to advocate for better outcomes. This principle became the foundation for every major advancement that followed. Lillian Wald expanded nursing beyond hospital walls with public health nursing. Mary Eliza Mahoney broke racial barriers as the first African American licensed nurse, opening doors for generations to follow. Mary Elizabeth Carnegie fought for quality education and racial recognition, becoming a Living Legend of the American Academy of Nursing.

Each had to navigate their own maze after feeling trapped by the limitations of their time.

The pattern continues today. Each of these historical moments share a common thread: a nurse identified a problem, refused to accept traditional definitions of success, and created a solution that expanded what nursing could accomplish. They didn't wait for permission. They saw a need, leveraged their unique know-how, and made lasting change.

What if the challenges you're facing today—the frustrations that brought you to this book—are the same stirrings that motivated every nursing pioneer before you?

Through thirteen chapters, you've discovered your peaks and valleys, explored many potential doors, and identified your unique know-how. You've learned that the "right" problems aren't the loudest ones—they're the ones that intersect your unique know-how with genuine needs your leaders can recognize and measure. You now understand that strategic thinking transforms trapped feelings into possibility. You've learned to reconnect with nature as your reset button. You've discovered that professional relationships are one of your most valuable navigation tools because they hold the extraordinary power to transform your experience from solitary struggle into collaborative breakthrough.

The physicians who trust your judgment, the colleagues who seek your guidance, the managers who value your perspective—these relationships don't just make your day better. They create the conditions where you can contribute in multiple dimensions. When you're known as someone who holds up honest mirrors, who extracts learning from difficult feedback, and who stays focused on what serves patients, you become someone people want to collaborate with across different roles and responsibilities. That reputation is what allows you to build something far more sustainable than a linear career path.

I want you to reconsider everything you've been told about career ladders in nursing. Ladders only go two directions—up or down—and that linear thinking is what leads to nurses feeling trapped. Instead, think of your bedside career as a diversified investment portfolio inside the maze. Just as a smart investor doesn't put everything into one stock, you don't bet everything on just one professional path. You increase your chances of success when you spread your energy across several categories. You might have 30% of your professional identity invested in precepting, 25% in clinical innovation, 20% in mentoring, 15% in specialized procedures, and 10% in unit leadership. When one area faces challenges, your other investments keep your career stable and growing. When one path narrows or hits a dead end, the others keep you moving forward. That's how you stay intentional in a maze that usually wears people down over time. Each category represents a different part of your professional success, and here's the best part: you get to decide which categories matter.

Traditional nursing success says climb to management or get another degree. Portfolio success says spread your bets, grow what works, and steadily increase your investment where you create the most value.

Traditional Nursing Success Says:

> ➤ Climb the ladder: bedside charge nurse supervisor manager director
> ➤ Get more degrees: BSN→MSN→DNP
> ➤ Leave the bedside as soon as possible
> ➤ More money equals more success
> ➤ Your title determines your value

Success Redefined Says:

> ➤ Build a portfolio: preceptor+innovator+consultant+bedside expert
> ➤ Develop deep expertise that makes you irreplaceable
> ➤ The bedside is where healthcare actually happens—own that power

> ➤ Success is measured in lives changed, systems improved, nurses retained

> ➤ Your impact determines your value

This kind of success requires courage. Follow the energy, not the title. It's easier to follow the prescribed path, to climb the visible ladder, to pursue achievements everyone recognizes. It takes guts to say, "My success looks different," and really mean it.

Discovering your unique know-how is where your journey to your unique purpose began. Your unique purpose is the end result: the clear understanding of how that know-how translates into meaningful work that's distinctly yours.

My Unique Know-How to Unique Purpose

I discovered that my unique know-how was this combination: foresight and clinical planning—I could look at a patient's picture and anticipate complications before they happened, organize my shift strategically, and assess my staff's capabilities and limitations very early in the shift when I was assigned the role of charge nurse. Foresight and clinical planning. What energizes me most is sharing new ideas and watching nurses execute effectively to achieve the outcomes we wanted.

And my perspective? I approached everything from a place of being overly prepared because I struggled early in my career—I became obsessive about note-taking and grouping information so I could work more efficiently.

For years, I thought that combination meant I was supposed to climb the traditional leadership ladder—become a supervisor, then a manager, and move up through the ranks. That's what leaders do, right?

But my unique purpose revealed something completely different. I stayed at the bedside on my own terms, launched a business, and now I write books and create resources that help nurses in my specialty find their confidence faster than I ever did. Today I have two income streams—bedside shifts when I want them and a company that energizes me in ways my clinical work alone never could.

Where Are You in the Journey to Unique Purpose?

You've Started the Process When:

- You can name 3-5 specific nursing skills you've developed
- You've identified at least one activity in your work that genuinely energizes you
- You're asking yourself "what makes me different?" instead of "why me?"

You Know You're Close to Your Unique Purpose When:

- You can clearly articulate what you're exceptionally good at (your skills)
- You know exactly what energizes you most in your work (your passion)
- You can explain what makes your approach different from other nurses (your perspective)

> ➤ You can describe in one sentence how these three things work together to create value

> ➤ You're making career decisions based on alignment with this purpose, not just escaping your feeling of being trapped at the bedside

The Proof: *You can now see opportunities you were blind to before—roles, projects, or paths that align perfectly with your unique combination of skills, passions, and perspective that you would have scrolled past or never even considered. What once looked like a confusing maze of options now has clear yeses and nos.*

You picked up this book because you felt trapped at the bedside. But that feeling wasn't about the bedside itself. I believe that feeling was the natural tension created when we attempt to achieve success using someone else's blueprint. Your unique purpose within bedside nursing isn't some hidden treasure waiting to be discovered. It's the path itself—the unique way you navigate challenges, the specific portfolio you build, the unique professional direction you follow.

The bedside needs nurses who refuse to see it as a trap. It needs nurses who recognize that the most important work in healthcare happens right there, in those moments between medication passes, in those insights that come from being present with patients day after day.

As you step into your next shift, you're not the same nurse who started this book. You understand that challenges aren't barriers blocking your path but your invitation to build something that never existed before. Every nurse who seems trapped is actually standing at the intersection of infinite possibilities. *The only difference between trapped and legendary is the decision to stop navigating with someone else's definition of success and start creating your own.*

Your unique career path doesn't require anyone's permission. It doesn't need to make sense to anyone but you. Your path doesn't need to follow any traditional trajectory. All it needs is for you to trust your compass, build your portfolio, and take the next step in the direction that feels like the best fit for you.

This is where the book ends, but where your best work begins. You now stand at a crossroad in the maze—two paths before you.

Path one: close this book, feel the inspiration wash over you for a week and slip back into the familiar patterns that brought you here.

Path two: decide right now, in this very moment, to take one strategic action this week toward your unique purpose.

What makes this extraordinary isn't your choice alone. It's the cascade that follows. The nurse who sees your courage finds her own. The problem you solve becomes the template another nurse desperately needs. Your refusal to shrink, to leave, to accept borrowed definitions of success—that refusal reverberates through every shift that follows. Legends aren't built in isolation.

They're built in the presence of others. Watching. Learning. Discovering that transformation is possible.

One strategic action. This week. That's the bridge between reading about change and becoming it. Success isn't about escaping the bedside—it's about transforming your experience of it.

What once held you captive now holds infinite possibility. Legends transform mazes into masterpieces.

You know your two paths. You know legends aren't born—they're made in mazes. So what will you build at the bedside that no one has ever built before?

That is your unique path. Now, my friend… go and build something beautiful!

WORKBOOK

A GUIDE TO DISCOVERING YOUR UNIQUE PURPOSE AND CREATING YOUR NEW PATH FORWARD

How to Use This Workbook

This workbook is designed to be your personal guide for discovering your unique purpose within bedside nursing. Each section builds on the previous one, creating a complete picture of who you are, what you're capable of, and how you can express your distinctive purpose within bedside nursing.

Instructions:

- ➢ Work through each section honestly and thoroughly
- ➢ Use this as an ongoing tool for career reflection and growth
- ➢ Share insights with trusted mentors or colleagues when appropriate

Chapter 1: Breaking Free Starts Here: Recognizing Your Starting Point

Reflection Exercise: Mapping Your Maze

What does your maze look like right now?

Describe your current situation in nursing - the walls you keep hitting, the paths that seem to lead nowhere:

____

____

____

____

When was the last time you felt like you were standing on a peak?

What made you feel strong, capable, and connected to your purpose?

When was the last time you felt like you were in a valley?

What made you feel overwhelmed, unsure, or disconnected?

What's one step you can take today to remind yourself that you're still moving, even if you can't see the exit?

Chapter 2: The Power to Pivot: Using Change to Break Free

Choose One Exercise That Resonates Most

Exercise 1: The Values Collision Map

Three moments of frustration/moral distress in your nursing career:

1. Situation: ___________________________________

    Core value being compromised: _____________________

2. Situation: ___________________________________

    Core value being compromised: _____________________

3. Situation: ___________________________________

    Core value being compromised: _____________________

Three moments when you felt most alive and authentic:

1. Situation: ___________________________________

    Value fully expressed: ___________________________

2. Situation: ___________________________________

    Value fully expressed: ________________________

3. Situation: ___________________________________

    Value fully expressed: ___________________________

Exercise 2: The Patient Story Mirror

Write the stories of two patients who impacted you most deeply:

Patient Story 1:

____

____

____

____

____

____

____

What did you learn about yourself through caring for them?

____

____

____

____

Patient Story 2:

____

____

____

____

____

____

What did you learn about yourself through caring for them?

____

____

____

What patterns do you see that point toward your authentic purpose?

____

____

____

Chapter 3: Peak Performance Clues: Your Sweet Spot at the Bedside

Identifying Your Natural Skills

What do your colleagues consistently ask you for help with?

1. ____

2. ____

3. ____

4. ____

5. ____

6. ____

7. ____

8. ____

9. ____

10. ____

What pattern do you notice in these requests?

____

____

____

____

____

When do you lose track of time at work? Describe a specific situation:

Chapter 4: The Valleys of Growth: Learning from the Low Points

Your Hardest Moment Reflection

What did that experience teach you about your strength?

____

____

____

____

How did you adapt in ways you didn't expect?

____

____

____

____

What part of you grew because of that struggle?

____

____

____

____

Chapter 5: The Mindset Reset:Your Daily Escape Mechanism

Since mastery over motion is often one of the first doors nurses need to walk through, let's explore what mastery looks like in the context of bedside nursing. It's not just about clinical skills—it's about becoming the kind of nurse who moves with clarity and intention under pressure.

The Seven Areas of Bedside Mastery

1. Time Awareness

Definition: Understanding how to pace your shift so nothing important gets dropped, even when priorities change unexpectedly. This includes learning to estimate how long tasks actually take and building realistic timelines for your day.

My Current Challenge:

____

____

____

____

____

____

____

2. Clinical Judgment

Definition: Developing the ability to recognize what's normal, what's changing, and what needs escalation before situations become urgent. This comes from experience combined with intentional reflection on patient outcomes.

An area where I need to trust my instincts more:

____

____

____

____

3. Task Prioritization

Definition: Making decisions based on patient safety and optimal outcomes, not just responding to whoever is asking the loudest or most persistently.

I struggle most with prioritizing when:

____

____

____

____

4. Workflow Strategy

Definition: Creating personal systems so you're not reinventing your approach every day. This includes developing routines for medication administration, documentation, and patient assessments that become second nature.

One routine I've developed that works well:

____

____

____

____

____

____

An area where I need a better system:

____

____

____

____

____

____

5. Emotional Regulation

Definition: Maintaining composure during chaotic situations so you can lead yourself and support others effectively. This skill is crucial for both patient safety and your own wellbeing.

My biggest emotional trigger at work is:

____

____

____

____

____

One technique I use (or want to try) to stay calm:

____

____

____

____

____

____

6. Boundary Management

Definition: Learning to say no to distractions and requests that don't align with your priorities or patient safety needs. This includes managing interruptions and maintaining focus on essential tasks.

I find it hardest to say no when:

____

____

____

____

____

____

A boundary I need to set or strengthen:

____

____

____

____

____

____

7. Self-Awareness

Definition: Recognizing when you're slipping into survival mode and knowing how to pull yourself back into intentional practice.

I know I'm in survival mode when:

____

____

____

____

To get back to a more intentional practice, I want to:

____

____

____

____

Your Daily Escape Mechanism

Which of these seven areas currently makes you feel most "trapped" at the bedside?

____

____

____

Which area, when mastered, would give you the greatest sense of freedom and control?

____

____

____

____

Thoughtful Question: If you focused on mastering just one of these seven areas, which one would change the way you move through the maze more than any other?

My answer: _________________________________

Why this area would be my daily escape mechanism:

____

____

____

____

____

____

Chapter 6: The Key to Breaking Out: Your Unique Purpose Within Bedside Nursing

What life experiences have shaped how you see healthcare?

____

____

____

____

____

____

How do these experiences help you connect with patients and families?

____

____

____

____

____

____

What do you see that other nurses might miss because of your unique perspective?

____

____

____

____

____

____

____

Define your purpose in one sentence: What specific problem can you uniquely solve? What value do you bring to the bedside that others don't?

"I am the nurse who..."

____

____

____

____

____

Chapter 7: Strategic Thinking for Trapped Nurses: Problem-Solving Your Way Out

Your Problem-Solving Style

What type of problems do you naturally gravitate toward solving on your floor?

\
\
\
\
\

What's one problem solving strategy you would like to try?

\
\
\
\
\

What's the first step you'll take to apply this new strategy?

What steps could you take to become genuinely expert in your chosen area of focus?

Chapter 8: The Ultimate Advantage: The Hidden Power Every Bedside Nurse Already Possesses

Your First Story: Write about the weirdest, most unexpected thing that happened during your shift that no one outside of nursing would believe. Every nurse has that one story—the bizarre patient request, the ridiculous family drama, the impossible situation you somehow handled, the moment that made you think "I can't make this stuff up." Write about yours.

Make it real. Make it yours. Make other nurses laugh, cringe, or shake their heads.

Write Here:

____

____

____

____

____

____

____

____

This is your starting point. Every powerful voice begins with one unforgettable moment.

Chapter 9: The Impact of Meeting the Right Person: A Connection that Can Change Your Path

Finding Your People

Based on your unique interests and strengths, what nursing communities align with your purpose?

Research and list 3-5 specific groups:

1. ____

2. ____

3. ____

4. ____

5. ____

Growing Your Tribe

Who in your professional life has inspired or challenged you?

____

____

____

____

____

____

Is there someone you've admired but haven't reached out to yet? What's stopping you?

What steps can you take this week to build or strengthen a professional connection?

If you could only implement five networking ideas from this chapter over the next 6 months, which five would create the most freedom in your career?

Networking Idea 1:

Networking Idea 2:

____

____

____

____

Networking Idea 3:

____

____

____

____

Networking Idea 4:

____

____

____

____

Networking Idea 5:

____

____

____

____

Chapter 10: One Step Outside: Breaking Free from Bedside Limitations

What's one outdoor space nearby where you can go to reset after a shift?

____

____

____

____

____

____

How can you build small nature breaks into your weekly or daily routine?

____

____

____

____

____

____

Chapter 10: The Master Key - Turning Know-How into Impact

Taking Action: Powerful Questions for your Strategic Obsession

Instructions: Understanding these principles intellectually is one thing; applying them to your specific situation requires honest self-reflection. Take some time to consider these questions, and don't rush your answers. The goal isn't to have everything figured out immediately, but to begin the process of intentional career development.

What aspect of your current job energizes you rather than drains you?

____

____

____

____

When do you feel most competent and confident in your abilities?

____

____

____

____

____

What type of problems do you naturally gravitate toward solving on your floor?

What steps could you take to become genuinely expert in your chosen area of focus?

Who could you learn from who has already developed expertise in this area?

What resources could help you go deeper?

What problems in your workplace align with your unique know-how?

How could you measure the impact of solving these problems?

Who are the decision-makers who would care about these improvements?

My Strategic Obsession:

My Solution Based Plan:

Have you found a new professional pathway? If so, what is it...

Chapter 12: The CEO Mindset: Becoming the CEO of Your Nursing Career

Think about your most challenging shift in the past month. List three specific situations where you made decisions, solved problems, or coordinated resources. For each situation, rewrite it using business language instead of nursing language.

If you had to present your nursing experience to a hospital board as qualifications for a leadership position, what would be your top three accomplishments? Write each accomplishment in terms of measurable impact: What problems did you solve? What outcomes did you improve? What resources do you manage effectively?

Chapter 13: The Professional Mirror: How Feedback Reflects Your Path to Excellence

Think about a piece of feedback you received in the last month that triggered a strong emotional reaction.

Step 1: Identify the Mirror Type Which type of feedback mirror was it? □ Appreciation Mirror (recognizing your impact) □ Coaching Mirror (showing growth opportunities) □ Evaluation Mirror (reflecting professional standards)

Step 2: Recognize Your Trigger What made this feedback difficult to hear? □ Competence Trigger (questioned your clinical knowledge) □ Care Trigger (suggested you weren't compassionate enough) □ Autonomy Trigger (felt controlling or micromanaging) □ Other:

Step 3: Mine for Gold Looking past how it was delivered, write one specific thing from this feedback that could help you better serve your patients:

____

____

____

____

____

Step 4: Your Action Step What's one small change you could make based on this insight?

____

____

____

____

____

Recall a time when you received valuable feedback from someone whose delivery was poor. Describe the situation:

____

____

____

____

The problematic delivery (tone, timing, setting, etc.):

____

____

____

The useful message hidden inside:

____

____

____

____

How this insight helped you improve your patient care:

____

____

____

Your takeaway: How can you remember to separate the messenger from the message in future feedback situations?

____

____

____

These activities help you practice extracting value from feedback regardless of how it's delivered, turning every reflection into navigation data for your nursing journey.

Chapter 14: Success Redefined: Considering Your Unique Career Path

Exercise 1: Redefine Your Success Metrics

You've been measuring your career against someone else's ruler. It's time to build your own.

Instructions: Write down the traditional success metrics you've been judging yourself against (promotions, degrees, salary increases, etc.). Next, consider your redefined success metrics. Success that matters to you.

Traditional Success Metrics: *Ex*. *"Getting my MSN"*

____

____

____

____

My Redefined Success Metrics: Ex. "Becoming the go-to expert for complex wounds"

____

____

____

____

____

____

____

____

____

____

____

____

____

Now answer these questions:

1. What would change in your daily work life if you measured success by your own metrics instead of traditional ones?

    ____

    ____

    ____

2. Who in your life might not understand or approve of your redefined success? How will you handle that?

    ____

    ____

    ____

____

3. Write a one-sentence declaration of your success: "I will consider my bedside career successful when ______________

____."

____

____

____

4. What evidence would prove to you that you're succeeding by your own definition? (Be specific—what would you see, feel, or experience?)

____

____

____

____

Exercise 2: Build Your Career Portfolio

Traditional career planning asks "What's your next step up the ladder?" This exercise asks something better: "What's your ideal professional mix?"

Instructions: Think of your bedside career as an investment portfolio where you allocate your professional energy across different areas. Using the framework below, assign percentages that total 100% based on where you want to invest your time and energy over the next 6-12 months.

My Career Portfolio:

> - Clinical Expertise (specialized skills, certifications, procedures): ______%

> - Mentoring/Precepting (developing other nurses): ______%

> - Innovation/Quality Improvement (improving systems and processes): ______%

> - Unit Leadership (informal influence, committee work): ______%

> - Education (teaching, presenting, contributing knowledge): ______%

> - Patient Advocacy (specialized patient populations, support): ______%

> - Other (define): __________________ ______%

> - Other (define): __________________ ______%

Total: 100%

Reflection Questions:

1. How does your current reality compare to your ideal portfolio? Where are the biggest gaps?

____

____

____

____

2. What's one concrete action you could take this month to shift your portfolio 5% closer to your ideal?

____

____

____

3. How would your job satisfaction change if your portfolio matched what you designed above?

____

____

____

____

Exercise 3: From Trapped to Legendary Action Plan

The difference between feeling trapped and becoming legendary is action. This exercise bridges that gap.

Part A: Your Compass Calibration

Look back through your previous chapter reflections. What patterns emerge about your:

- ➢ Peak moments (when you feel most alive at work):
- ➢ Natural strengths (what comes easily to you):
- ➢ Deep frustrations (what drains you most):
- ➢ Unique perspective (what you see that others miss):

Part B: Your Next-Step Blueprint

Based on your compass above, identify three specific moves you can make:

1. Within the next 30 days:

- ➤ Action:
- ➤ Why this matters to my redefined success:
- ➤ Support/resources I need:

2. Within the next 90 days:

- ➤ Action:
- ➤ Why this matters to my redefined success:
- ➤ Support/resources I need:

3. Within the next 6 months:

- ➤ Action:
- ➤ Why this matters to my redefined success:
- ➤ Support/resources I need:

Part C: Your Declaration

Complete this statement and write it somewhere you'll see it regularly:

"I refuse to see the bedside as a trap because ____________________ ______________________________. The most important work in healthcare happens right here, and my unique contribution is ______________________________. I'm building something beautiful by ______________________________."

Final Reflection:

Six months from now, what will be different about your bedside career? Be specific and bold. This is your vision—make it count.